Yoga For Low Back And Hip Health

Gentle and Restorative Yoga to relieve chronic low back, hip and sciatic nerve pain

Cyndi Roberts, E-RYT 200

Copyright © 2016 Cyndi Roberts
All rights reserved.
ISBN: 1530550181
ISBN-13: 978-1530550180

DEDICATION

This book was written from a lifetime of experience and I have many people to dedicate it to:

- My family, especially my husband. Without the unconditional love and support, this book wouldn't have manifested. It's a true creation of love, learning, dedication and hard work.
- My amazing clients that are my inspiration and also my teachers. We often teach what we need to learn and they are always there to remind me what I need to get back home.
- The wonderful healers and teachers that I have had the privilege of working with along my path. In many different ways, with many unique experiences, they have opened my eyes, ears and heart to see, hear and feel what I needed most to heal.
- All of the people in the world that live with chronic back and hip pain that are looking for another way back to well-being and health, that doesn't include surgery or drugs.

CONTENTS

DEDICATION	iii
CONTENTS	v
INTRODUCTION	i
What causes back pain?	3
What causes low back pain?	5
The six directions of the spine	6
What causes irritation to the sciatic nerve?	7
What are the chakra systems?	9
HOW TO USE THIS BOOK	11
ABOUT ME	15
My life with chronic pain	19
Yoga teaching certifications	21
YOGA PROPS	23
HOW TO GET MAXIMUM BENEFIT FROM THE POSES AND STRETCHES IN THIS BOOK	23
Bolster	24
Mexican Blanket	25
Yoga Block	28
Yoga Strap	29
Eye Pillow (optional)	29
CHAPTER ONE	31
CORE STRENGTHENING YOGA POSES	31
Bent Leg Abs with Block	33
Bent Leg Twisting Abs with Block	35
Bicycle Abs	38
Pelvic Tilts	41
Plank Pose	44
Table Extensions	46
CHAPTER TWO	49
RESTORATIVE YOGA POSE INSTRUCTION	49
Belly Down ½ Frog	50
Reclined ½ Crescent	52

Reclined Leg Rest	54
Supported Belly Down Twist	56
Supported Belly Down Twist (Extended Leg Variation)	60
Supported Bridge With Bent Legs	62
Supported Child's Pose	64
Supported Final Relaxation	66
Supported ½ Moon	69
Supported Inversion	75
Side Lying Pose	78
Supported Pigeon Pose	80
Supported Reclining Pose	83
Supported Resting Butterfly	86

CHAPTER THREE   **89**
  GENTLE YOGA POSE INSTRUCTION   **89**

Cat/Cow Tilts	90
Child's Pose	92
Downward Facing Dog	95
Hip Circles	97
Low Lunge Hands On Thigh	99
Modified Downward Facing Dog	102
Reclined Knee Down Twist	104
Reclined Knee Hug (both knees)	106
Reclined Knee Hug (one knee)	108
Reclined Pigeon Pose	110
Reclined Three Part Hamstring Stretch	113
Reclined Three Part Hamstring Stretch: Part One	114
Reclined Three Part Hamstring Stretch: Part Two	115
Reclined Three Part Hamstring Stretch: Part Three	116
Seated Forward Fold	118
Seated Pigeon With Half Hero	121
Seated Side Bend	127
Seated Twist	130
Side Lying Quad Stretch	132
Table Pose	134
Four Part Pigeon	136
Four Part Pigeon: Part One	137
Four Part Pigeon: Part Two	138

Four Part Pigeon: Part Three   139
Four Part Pigeon: Part Four   140

CHAPTER FOUR   141
YOGA SEQUENCES   141

Sequence #1
Ease Low Back Pain
Gentle Yoga (short sequence)   142

Sequence #2
Ease Low Back Pain
Gentle Yoga (long sequence)   145

Sequence #3
Ease Low Back Pain
Restorative Yoga (short sequence)   151

Sequence #4
Ease Low Back Pain
Restorative Yoga (long sequence)   154

Sequence #5
Ease Hip Tension
Gentle Yoga (short sequence)   157

Sequence #6
Ease Hip Tension
Gentle Yoga (long sequence)   161

Sequence #7
Ease Hip Tension
Restorative Yoga (short sequence)   167

Sequence #8
Ease Hip Tension
Restorative Yoga (long sequence)   170

Sequence #9
Sequence for Piriformis Syndrome/Sciatic Nerve Pain
Gentle and Restorative Yoga (short sequence)   174

Sequence #10
Sequence for Piriformis Syndrome/Sciatic Nerve Pain
Gentle and Restorative Yoga (long sequence)   178

Sequence #11
Sequence for Core Strength Gentle and Restorative Yoga (short sequence)   182

Sequence #12
Sequence for Core Strength
Gentle and Restorative Yoga (short sequence)   184

Sequence #13
Sequence for Core Strength
Gentle and Restorative Yoga (long sequence)   188

Sequence #14
Sequence for Core Strength
Gentle and Restorative Yoga (long sequence)   192

Sequence #15
Sequence for Core Strength
Gentle and Restorative Yoga (long sequence)   195

This book was written to help you increase your level of health, awareness and well-being. The instruction, information and advice presented by me are in no way meant to be a substitute for counseling from your doctor. **Please consult your doctor before beginning this program or any other healthcare program.**

INTRODUCTION

Congratulations – you are one step closer to healthy and happy back and hips! The suggested poses and sequences in this book are ideal for beginners as well as advanced yogis. You will see the most benefit by practicing the poses and sequences consistently, three to four times per week.

When I transitioned from teaching group yoga classes to teaching one-on-one yoga sessions in 2012, I was able to more effectively help my students find the yoga that was right for their bodies. I had the opportunity to focus on specific health issues and use yoga as a way to ease symptoms. I knew this is what I was meant to teach. Expanding my knowledge of anatomy and movement has helped me serve my clients more effectively.

Low back, hip and sciatic nerve pain are some of the most common issues that I have seen and worked with as my client base has expanded. Not only have my clients found relief, but I have as well.

Seeing the continued positive results within myself and my clients, I documented some of my favorite restorative yoga postures, gentle stretches and sequences in this book to share with you.

You'll find detailed instruction and over three-hundred high resolution photos to assist you safely through your practice. I offer modifications and variations of each pose to ensure you find what is right for you and your body.

In addition, there is information about the seven chakras systems that this book addresses. I'll provide detailed information about each energy system and the corresponding poses in Chapter Two: Restorative Yoga Instruction. (More information about the chakra system is provided on page nine.)

Chronic low back pain is a health issue that I have been working with personally since 2001. Prior to discovering yoga in 2009, I tried everything to relieve the chronic pain I lived with. Beginning a regular yoga practice in 2009 – and remaining committed to it – provided the relief that I was so desperately seeking.

I discovered that through daily practice, my chronic back pain disappeared. Stretching was the answer to my distress. Passionately and curiously, I dove deeply into the study of yoga, anatomy, pranayama (breathing exercises), yoga nidra, relaxation and spirituality. I knew within my being that I had to learn and teach.

When I was pregnant with my son in 2014, I experienced daily sciatic nerve pain toward the end of my pregnancy. I used my practice – modifying for pregnancy of course – to relieve the pain down my leg and in my foot.

Since the birth of my son, I occasionally experience sciatic pain, especially on days when I sit for too long. I always come back to my yoga and find relief immediately. I know you will too.

WHAT CAUSES BACK PAIN?

The most common causes of pain in the back body are tight muscles, in the back, pelvis, hips and hamstrings. These tight muscles are most often caused by improper alignment, poor posture or sitting or standing for long hours. Of course, there may be other issues – especially in extreme cases – where unhealthy discs are the cause. **Describe your symptoms to your doctor and have an MRI to be sure if you are experiencing extreme pain.**

However, if there are no signs of major injury, the cause of your pain may simply be tight muscles. If it is a muscular issue, no drugs or surgery are required for you to get relief. Isn't that exciting to know!? Isn't that a relief!? I personally feel it's truly empowering to know that I'm in control of my health and that I can significantly reduce my pain levels without drugs or surgery. The guided instruction and safe postures carefully chosen for this book can be a starting point to take responsibility for your health so you too can experience true holistic healing.

If you practice these stretches and poses mindfully and do not feel pain, that is a good sign from the body that you aren't hurting anything. Sure, there may be times when you feel sensation, ranging from a gentle stretch to an intense sensation, but keep in mind, sensation is much different than pain.

Sensation and pain both exist to help you become aware of what the body is trying to tell you. Feeling pain is a way the body communicates danger. Feeling sensation is a sign the body is tense and it needs to soften and let go. Practicing the poses and gentle stretches in this book will help you tune into that voice, listen and connect to the wisdom that lies within. You will know what is right for *your* body as you regularly practice and tune in. Your body is ultimately your teacher.

Be aware of tingling, numbness, burning, sharp or electric pain as you move through each of the poses and stretches. Those are important signs from the body to back off or come out of the pose.

If you are aware of the stretching sensation, it most likely means that you are stretching a tight place. It's our practice to breathe with those sensations and soften with them. The body will open when it is ready and the breath encourages and supports the muscles as they let go of built up tension and stress. Soft body, soft mind. Soft mind, soft body.

As I mentioned before, the poses and stretches in this book were carefully chosen and are safe and gentle. If something hurts or doesn't feel right, don't practice it or use a modification. This book is merely a guide. Your body will ultimately show you the way to healing, so be committed, be quiet and listen.

WHAT CAUSES LOW BACK PAIN?

Though you may not be entirely sure of what is causing your low back pain (**consult your doctor in cases of extreme pain**), gentle stretching is useful to relieve built-up tension and stress in the muscles. Gentle stretching also keeps the joints healthy and flexible. Regular stretching rebuilds strength in weak muscles and increases flexibility. Healthy joints and flexible muscles contribute to a body free from stiffness and common aches and pains.

According to The Mayo Clinic, "Back pain is one of the most common reasons people go to the doctor or miss work and a leading cause of disability worldwide." In most cases, increased amounts of sitting combined with a sedentary lifestyle, the body – especially the low back – becomes tight and inflexible. This tightness creates aches and pains in the low back and hip area. Fortunately, gentle movements relieve the stiffness and pain when practiced regularly.

One way to address the pain is by focusing on the muscle groups in the back and hips. The spine connects these muscles together and a healthy spine is able to move in six directions. Moving the spine in all six directions relieves tension and discomfort in all the muscles of the back body and hips, while increasing flexibility in the joints.

Practicing the yoga poses and stretches in this book will reduce stress

in the spine, especially from prolonged sitting at the office or driving. Stiffness in the front and side bodies will also be relieved, creating flexibility in the spine and strengthening weaker muscles.
Improving the health of the spine by bringing movement to the joints relieves stagnation and increases synovial fluid, which lubricates the joints. Lubricated joints are less prone to injury or pain.

THE SIX DIRECTIONS OF THE SPINE

The six directions of the spine include: forward bends, back bends, lateral movements (right/left), and twisting motions (right/left).

These movements are beneficial for a variety of reasons:

FORWARD BENDS
- Create length and space in the spine, countering compression between the disks
- Gently stretch out tight muscles in the back body
- Soothing and calming to the nervous system, reducing stress and anxiety
- Deep, slow breaths provide a gentle massage for abdominal organs which stimulate blood flow to digestive organs, thereby increasing organ function

BACKBENDS
- Elevate low moods and relieve sadness and depression
- Soften and open a compressed and tight front body, countering forward-rolling shoulders
- Open the heart center, chest, lungs, shoulders and hip flexors
- Improve breathing function by gently stretching the diaphragm
- Warm up the spine and promote flexibility

LATERAL MOVEMENTS/SIDE BENDS (RIGHT/LEFT)
- Lengthen the muscles between the ribs and pelvis (including parts of the low back and hips)
- Increase flexibility and circulation in the muscles of the ribs, pelvis, hips and spine
- Open the side body, rib cage and breathing muscles, which expand the lungs for easier breathing
- Loosen resistance in the spine and torso

TWISTS (RIGHT/LEFT)
- Improve mobility between the joints of the spine
- Gently stretch and maintain natural mobility in the spine
- Decompress the vertebrae and allow energy to flow more freely
- The squeeze and soak action of the organs when twisting is a way to detox and release stagnation and toxins
- Deep, slow breaths provide a gentle massage for abdominal organs, which stimulates blood flow to digestive organs, thereby improving organ function

While practicing the appropriate poses in this book, you naturally balance the over-stretched and under-stretched muscles of the lumbar region, bringing the pelvis back to neutral, taking the pressure off the low back. By both stretching and/or slackening the muscle imbalances in the low back and pelvis area relieves strain in the muscles. Muscle imbalances are released and low back and hip pain are relieved.

WHAT CAUSES IRRITATION TO THE SCIATIC NERVE?
You may not be exactly sure what causes sciatic pain (nerve pain down the leg), but yoga can help greatly if a tight muscle is to blame.

Consult your doctor in cases of extreme pain and have an MRI to check for a disk issue.

Sciatic pain most commonly occurs in one leg. It starts in the low back or buttocks and radiates down the back of the leg, and in some cases, into the foot. Some may describe the pain as sharp, searing or burning and standing or sitting for long periods of time may worsen the pain. Some women may experience it only during pregnancy as the weight of baby increases, as I did.

If you are experiencing pain in mid-lower back, tingling, burning, numbness or electro-shocks down the length of the leg, these can be signs of a more serious issue – a herniated disc – **and you should schedule an appointment with your doctor for an MRI.**

However, if you aren't experiencing these extreme symptoms, you may be suffering from piriformis syndrome and stretching tight muscles regularly will relieve the pain you are feeling.

The small but significant muscle deep within the hip called the piriformis (used to turn the hip out) has a nerve – the sciatic nerve – running through it. When tension builds up within this particular muscle, it compresses and irritates the nerve, creating obvious and sometimes intolerable pain.

Releasing hip structure and creating traction with gentle, regular stretching, takes pressure off the nerve. This may be all you need to manage and ease the pain. Additionally, by resting tightened muscles and bringing the pelvic area back into alignment you'll ease tension, pain and discomfort in the hip, buttocks and down the leg.

There is a way to feel better and find relief from piriformis syndrome and sciatic nerve pain without drugs or surgery. This book can show you how.

WHAT ARE THE CHAKRA SYSTEMS?

The human body is matter and form but it is also energy. The seven chakras are the energy centers in the body that are most commonly talked about, but there are actually one-hundred and fourteen energy centers in the body. They're all interconnected throughout our being, across the mid-line and extending out to shoulders, hands, fingers and feet.

This book focuses on the seven chakras along the mid-line of the body. These "wheels" of energy radiate from the nerve endings of the spinal column and sit on top of one another from the tailbone to the crown of the head.

They coincide with basic states of consciousness, personality structures, coping mechanisms and emotions. Chakras are energy, much like feelings and thoughts. Each color of the rainbow is represented with each chakra. Together and in balance, this union of the colors of the rainbow unites our minds, bodies and spirits.

In yogic philosophy, our Kundalini energy starts out at the base of the spine, representing either a goddess or sleeping serpent waiting to be awakened. When the Kundalini energy is awakened, she dances through the rainbow chakras, bringing color and healing to our stagnant and stuck black and white worlds of conformity and suffering.

When this energy is flowing freely, this dance of transformation connects the gap between matter and consciousness. The self takes a journey through the wheels of the chakra rainbow, reconnecting to and reclaiming its true divine nature.

Healing the chakras connects us to spiritual wealth, which is within all of us. Balancing the chakra centers releases old patterns in the body that no longer serve us, as we wake to a more vibrant state of being and presence.

When we balance the chakras, energy flows freely through each point, connecting us to our essence, our bodies, one another, our true divine nature and ultimately, the universe. Balanced chakra energies heal aches, discomfort and pain caused by stagnation in the mind, body and spirit.

HOW TO USE THIS BOOK

You will find the names, safe guided instruction and high resolution photos for each core strengthening yoga poses in Chapter One. Chapters Two includes restorative yoga postures and Chapter Three contains gentle yoga postures. Chapter Four provides original sequences, both long and short, with pictures and names in the order of the suggested sequence. There are over three-hundred high resolution photos to guide you!

Short sequences can range from twenty to forty minutes and the long sequences can range from an hour to ninety minutes. If you find that you want to practice more than twenty minutes, after completing a short sequence, choose another short sequence to practice or simply extend the length of one or two restorative poses, including supported final relaxation.

As you practice the sequences, I suggest you to go back to the previous chapters to learn the specific instruction for each pose. Make safety a priority. Practicing proper alignment of each pose will ensure you receive the most benefit.

As you practice and connect inward, find the first place of resistance in the body when stretching. Connect with the sensations in the body and breathe into the stretch. As the breath deepens and the body opens, you may find that you can stretch deeper, as the muscle tension begins to dissipate. As you stay and breathe with sensation, the body will gently open at its own rate. Be sure to listen to the body and not force a stretch.

If you are feeling pain, you may have gone too deep into the stretch and I urge you to ease out of the deep stretch or stop altogether. Remember, *your* body is your best teacher. Listen to what it has to say. These sequences are designed to gently stretch and de-stress the back, hips and legs – at no time is experiencing pain acceptable.

You want to be as comfortable as possible, especially when practicing the restorative postures. Feeling comfortable will allow relaxation and release. If you are not comfortable, the body will hold on, tighten and feel stressed, keeping you stuck in fight or flight mode. Fight or flight mode is the opposite of the relaxation response. Fight or flight mode creates stress and imbalances in the body. Relaxation mode brings healing and relief.

Find a quiet place with no distractions and journey within. Give yourself the gift of setting aside this sacred time to heal and let go.

Keep in mind that true healing comes from within, with a willingness to feel, without turning away. It is only when we drop resistance to feeling and become curious about what we are feeling, we begin to heal. Safely allowing and enduring our inner state with awareness and compassion is truly finding peace. Feeling allows relaxation. Relaxation allows healing.

It is normal to find yourself unable to relax, especially if you are new to the practice. Remember that if you are finding it difficult to let go, your body is conditioned to fight or flight mode and relaxation will be a gradual transition. Have compassion for where you are on your journey and give yourself the space to grow and soften.

I encourage you to compassionately discover sensation and feel it. Take time to get to know your body and the difference between pain and sensation. Be gentle with yourself and practice mindful movements at all times. Use this time to connect to and appreciate your physical body and breath. The body possesses an innate wisdom. Within each of us is our unique path to healing.

Spend time looking inward and unlock the wisdom of the body. Discover your unique path to feeling better, health, vitality and well-being. Be mindful of limitations and modifications that need to be made as you practice.

Included in the instruction are the appropriate props to use with each posture. Reference the suggested blanket folds in the "Yoga Props" section of the book.

If you are new to yoga, you may feel sore after practicing. This is normal and a good sign that you are getting things moving. Be sure to drink plenty of water to re-hydrate the tissues and muscles. Water not only re-hydrates but also flushes out toxins and waste.

I would again like to congratulate you on your choice to be responsible for your health. As someone that struggled with health issues, addiction and even faced death, I understand how uncomfortable you may feel if you are starting something new.

Keep in mind that you are not alone. Change happens outside of your comfort zone. It's never easy, but always worth it, especially if you are ready for lasting change that will allow you to blossom into the best version of yourself. Change happens with consistent small steps. One practice at a time, one breath at a time.

How healthy or unhealthy you are is something that is always in your hands. Regular practice will provide relief and well-being. Please contact me at Cyndi@yogawithcr.com, if you have any questions or check out my website, yogawithcr.com, for more information.

May you walk with peace, Namaste.

ABOUT ME

CYNDI ROBERTS

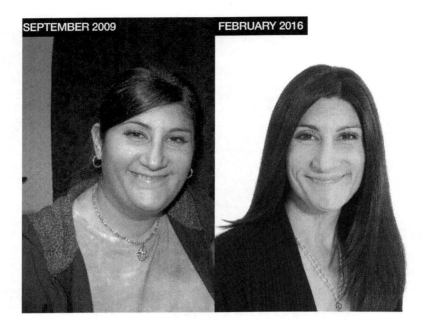

Life is something to celebrate and enjoy, not dread or fear. We all deserve to be happy and healthy. Though we all have a unique purpose, we are all connected. Through the practices of yoga, meditation and spirituality, I have found health, relief, lasting peace and happiness and I hope to help you do the same.

On the brink of death, I discovered life. There was a time when I was hopelessly lost in the dark, suffering and in pain. I was trapped in the despair of depression and the crippling grip of anxiety, with a prescription in my hand as the only option to feel better. For twelve long years I believed that *was* the only option and repeatedly trusted doctors' advice, never once questioning their decisions.

I was diagnosed with severe depression and anxiety disorder at the age of eighteen and put on prescription medication, from which I quickly began to experience side effects. Shortly after, I was misdiagnosed with bipolar disorder.

Like so many who are misdiagnosed, I was put on a cocktail of medications and lost in the system, given no other alternative – except for talk therapy – to feel better.

Side effects of the medications only made my state of mind and physical health deteriorate. I developed addictions to cigarettes, food, shopping, drugs and alcohol. I was searching for anything to free me from the hell I was trapped in. I was desperate for relief. I felt as though I was a victim to my circumstances and believed my diagnosis defined me.

Fast forward to 2009, when I was thirty years old. I was eighty pounds overweight, had countless addictions and was suicidally depressed. I was experiencing daily chronic pain, panic attacks so intense I could not leave the house, and facing liver failure, diabetes and death.

My naturopathic doctor performed blood tests to get a baseline of my health and the results were dismal. He informed me that my liver enzymes were equivalent to what he sees in sixty-year old lifelong alcoholics, and that I had about six months to live before my liver shut down completely.

I had officially hit "rock bottom" and was faced with a choice: to give up or fight. That day – the day I faced my own mortality – was the day I questioned everything. I realized it was up to me – and only me – to save my life. I needed to take responsibility for my health and not give my power away to doctors or blindly trust what they had to say.

At this point I realized that Western medicine had failed me and I had to find another way. I wondered if there was more to life than my misery, suffering and pain. I wondered if there would ever be a day that I felt happy to be alive, rather than trying to escape or fantasize about death.

I knew I had to start by safely getting off of my current medications. I spoke with my prescribing doctor who dismissed the blood tests and refused to help. After that, I spoke to more than thirty doctors trying to find one who was willing to help me safely get off the dozen medications I was on. Finally, number thirty-eight said yes.

The painful journey of detox began and I immersed myself in my artwork, exercise, nature, nutrition, the practices of yoga, meditation and the study of spiritual teachings that helped me take back control of my life.

With a lot of hard work, courage and dedication, I did it. I regained my health. As I write this book at the beginning of 2016, I am enjoying optimal health: eighty pounds lighter, free of pharmaceutical medications, addictions, severe depression, crippling anxiety and chronic pain.

Moment by moment, I choose life on my terms instead of waiting for the quick fix or the magic pill. I choose life without clouded judgment or the fog of medication or addictions like I once did. I found true peace and health by making a connection within.

I took responsibility for myself and stopped living as a victim, blaming others, and giving my power away. I stopped looking for others to "fix" or "complete" me. I stopped looking for others' approval and I faced my deepest fears and heartaches.

I also found healthy solutions that made sense for me. I began to question what was right for me and my healing. I took back control of my health and empowered myself with knowledge. Making a connection to my body, practicing mindfulness and awareness of the present moment dissolved my anxiety and depression.

For me, yoga is not a gimmick. Exercise and meditation aren't fads – these practices helped saved my life and have become an inextricable part of my daily routine. I'm not on the newest diet – I make healthy food choices one meal at a time and care about what I put in my body and mind.

These practices have become the cornerstones of my health. They allow me a life that's happy, healthy and balanced – a life that doctors said would never be possible without medication. These practices aren't new; they have been working for thousands of years, but we have become a disconnected society. Reconnecting saved my life.

Along with my diet, these practices play a major role in managing my moods, my state of mind and my physical health. I now have the strength to feel, the courage to take responsibility for my thoughts and actions and live my life for me.

I live what I teach and am a genuine person. I take pride in bringing something different to my students. I share insights gathered through lived experience and knowledge gained from continued study at trainings and workshops, as well as my ever-growing library of books.

Poses and stretches are only the tip of the iceberg that is yoga. As my personal practice deepens, I learn more about yoga as a way of life and discover the depth of what yoga truly means. It is my passion to discover those depths and apply it to modern day living. It is my passion to share and teach, helping others reclaim their health through yoga.

MY LIFE WITH CHRONIC PAIN

Having survived a near fatal car accident in 2001, my journey of living with chronic low back pain began. I tried everything to find relief, including using steroids, cortisol injections, pain killers (which I ultimately developed an addiction to) and regular physical therapy.

It wasn't until I started to detox from the numbing medications and started practicing yoga regularly in 2009 that I experienced relief. As the numbing effects of the medications wore off, the awareness of my low back pain became prevalent. I moved slowly, did what I could and stayed committed to my practice. Within a few months, I felt a drastic improvement.

Going from feeling chronic pain, achy, stiff and sore to feeling relief – without drugs or surgery – was nothing short of a miracle.

Nothing has helped the way yoga has. I no longer suffer from chronic low back pain and don't need medications or injections to numb the pain. I ultimately realized that my body was trying to tell me something. By taking medications, I was silencing my body. I was ignoring the inner wisdom and getting worse day by day.

My regular yoga practice allowed me to tune into what my body was saying, rather than silencing it. My continued dedication to my practice brings me health, relief, clarity and ease.

My hope is for my yoga students to develop this deep connection with their bodies and what they feel, rather than a connection to their heads and what they think. Pain and tension in the body are worsened when the mind is focused on negativity and stress. I want my students to be able to tune into the wisdom of the body, just as I did, to find their way back to well-being and health.

When we quiet the mind, the wisdom of the body prevails. Regular meditation, stretching, deep breathing and practicing positive affirmations are proven ways to reduce noise and negativity in the mind. When negative thoughts dissolve, so does tension in the body.

There is a unique connection between the mind and body. What we think, we feel. What we feel, we think. When dealing with pain, we have to look at that mind-body connection and address negative thinking about pain.

We must also look at whether we feel like victims in life. Does life happen *to* us or do we feel empowered, like we are active participants in our lives? Do we give away our power by blaming others for the circumstances of our life, or are we creators of our reality? Believe it or not, each viewpoint has a very different effect on pain and how it does or doesn't manifest in our bodies.

We must also ask if we are willing to feel or if we're avoiding feeling. What we resist persists, including pain. Liberation comes from feeling.

I know from my personal experience and ongoing work with my clients that properly and safely stretching away tension will have a profound effect on your life.

What would your life look like, not having to live with chronic pain, stiffness, soreness or aches and pains every day?

Yoga is proven to reduce stress levels and anxiety, while improving circulation and immune and organ function. Regularly practicing the yoga poses and stretches in this book will help you find the relief from low back, hip and sciatic nerve pain that you have been searching for, without drugs or surgery.

YOGA TEACHING CERTIFICATIONS

- E-RYT 200 (registered 200 hour Yoga Instructor through Yoga Alliance)
- Certified Therapeutic Yoga Instructor
- Certified Pranakriya Prenatal Yoga Instructor
- Certified Level I Reiki Master

YOGA PROPS

HOW TO GET MAXIMUM BENEFIT FROM THE POSES AND STRETCHES IN THIS BOOK

There are four basic yoga props you will need to get maximum benefit from the restorative postures and gentle stretches suggested in this book. The fifth prop is optional to maximize relaxation. Props are a wonderful addition to any yogi's practice and encourage safe surrender. They are versatile and useful, and not only for beginners.

BOLSTER

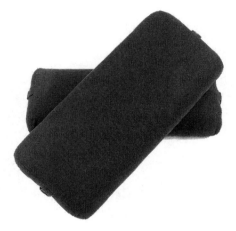

Bolster (25x12x6 inches)

Using a bolster while practicing is deeply supportive and allows you the space to let go and relax. In the state of relaxation, you become united with self, the present moment, mindfulness and the body naturally heals. I have used every size bolster in my personal practice and with clients. I found that the bolsters that measure 25 x 12 x 6 inches are the most versatile and comfortable. They reduce the risk of over-stretching and are most helpful with proper alignment and relaxation.

MEXICAN BLANKET

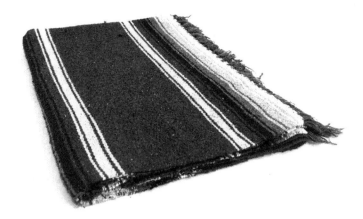

Large rectangle fold

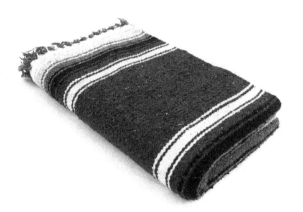

Small rectangle fold

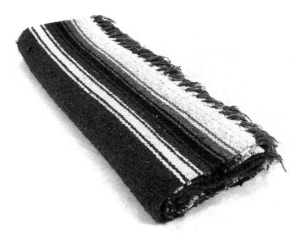

Long rectangle fold

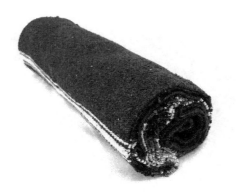

Blanket roll

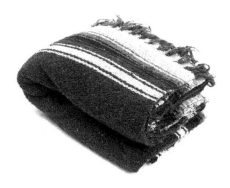

Square fold

Mexican blankets are an absolute must-have yoga prop, in my opinion. They are so versatile and can be folded or rolled in a variety of ways to support your practice. In addition, two or three blankets (long rectangle fold) can be used together to make the shape of a bolster or they can be used instead of blocks (square fold).

They are easy to wash in a regular washing machine and do well in the dryer. They are easy to maintain, withstand many washings and get softer with each wash. Blankets support the body in a variety of ways to help enhance certain poses, keep you comfortable in longer holds and help support proper alignment. They're also perfect to cover up with to keep warm or use for picnics.

YOGA BLOCK

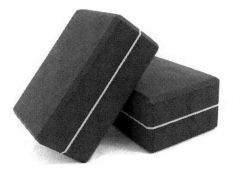

Foam yoga block (9x6x4 inches)

Yoga blocks are used for support to deepen postures and help with proper alignment. In most cases, the use of blocks can help you hold poses more comfortably and for longer periods of time, allowing the body to open in a safer way. Blocks are helpful for balance and to develop flexibility. There are three different materials to choose from.

Wood blocks are hollow, hard and heavy. Depending on the kind of wood they are made with, they may be unstable and slip when placed on a hardwood floor. Cork blocks are softer than wood and most eco-friendly. However, they absorb odors over time and have a tendency to crumble and dent the more they are used.

The yoga blocks in the above photo are foam, measuring 9x6x4 inches. Foam blocks are the least expensive option. Foam blocks without the stripe are soft and not as sturdy so I always choose the blocks with the stripe for more durability. They are also lightweight, easy to store and easy to clean. I recommend using foam blocks and prefer to use them when I practice and teach.

YOGA STRAP

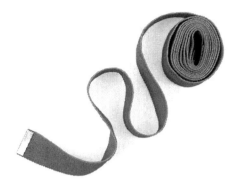

Yoga strap (8 feet)

Yoga straps are perfect props when you need to stretch limbs that you are unable to reach. They act as an extension of the arms so you can practice proper alignment and receive the most benefit of the stretch, even though your flexibility may not be where you want it. A yoga strap can also assist you with holding certain poses longer. Straps come in several lengths; 6 foot, 8 foot, or 10 foot. I am 5'8" and find that the 8 foot strap works perfectly for me.

EYE PILLOW (OPTIONAL)

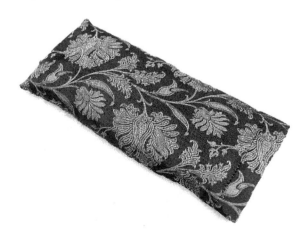

Eyepillow (optional)

Eye pillows are a wonderful addition for your restorative practice if you are looking to soothe the eyes and release tension in the forehead and the brow. An eye pillow is also useful to block out light and provide weight on the face for a deep state of relaxation and rest. Some eye pillows are scented, which can have additional healing and calming affects on your practice (specifically lavender scent).

CHAPTER ONE

CORE STRENGTHENING YOGA POSES

As we have discussed, back pain can be caused by many issues, including bad posture, straining a muscle when bending and lifting, or from a soft tissue injury. A natural deterioration of the spine and muscles from aging or weak core and back muscles could also be to blame.

The back and core muscles support the torso and the spine. The torso is the very center of our bodies (along with the hips), while the spine is the supporting frame for the back. Connecting the front body to the back body throughout these areas is an intricate system of muscles and ligaments.

When these muscles aren't strengthened or cared for, strength and stability are lost in the torso and spine. This lack of stability puts increased stress on the muscles of the spine that hold the body upright and that are used for movement. With lack of stability comes lack of balance and back injury and back pain become more likely. Strengthening the core means strengthening the spine and improving posture and structure. A strong core assists the spine and can relieve discomfort and pain in the back.

Practicing these core strengthening yoga poses will take the pressure off the spine and have your back stronger in no time. A strong core means a more balanced body.

BENT LEG ABS WITH BLOCK

This core strengthening pose is a gentle and safe way to heat up and engage the middle of the abdominal muscles. Having the legs bent in this pose is less strain on an already tight back. (For more intensity, lengthen both legs toward sky, pressing out through the toes.)

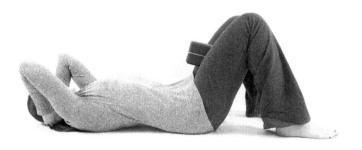

Bent Leg Abs with Block (inhale, hold breath, squeeze block, curl tailbone)

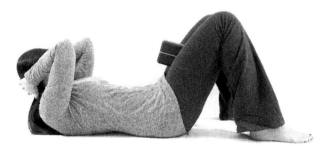

Bent Leg Abs with Block (exhale, lift head and shoulders off the earth)

INSTRUCTION

- Lie flat on your back with knees bent and feet hips width apart. Feel free to use a blanket support (long rectangle fold) under the head.
- Place a yoga block (the middle thickness) between the thighs.
- Interlace the hands behind the head, drawing the elbows in close together.
- Keep head and shoulders on the earth as you inhale.

- Hold the breath, squeeze the block, curl the tailbone.
- Exhale, lift head and shoulders off the earth, pull navel down to the spine.
- Inhale, head and shoulders down.
- Hold breath, squeeze block, curl tailbone.
- Exhale head and shoulders up, pull navel down.
- Repeat for 10 rounds.
- To release: remove the block and rest the hands on the belly. Take 4-5 long belly breaths while resting the knees together.
- Practice 2 more rounds, pausing between each round for belly breaths.

BENT LEG TWISTING ABS WITH BLOCK

This pose is a variation of Bent Leg Abs with Block but targets the side abdominals with its twisting action. Keeping the legs bent, again, keeps strain off already tight back muscles. (For more intensity, lift the feet off the earth, bending the legs to a ninety degree angle, stacking the knees over the hips. With each twist, straighten the opposite leg, twisting toward bent right knee as left leg straightens.)

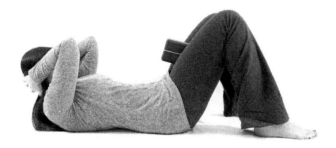

Bent Leg Twisting Abs with Block (inhale, head and shoulders off the earth)

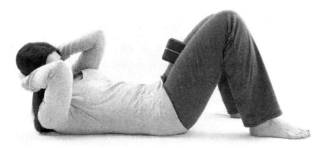

Bent Leg Twisting Abs with Block (exhale, twist to the right)

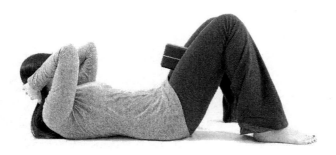

Bent Leg Twisting Abs with Block (inhale, head and shoulders back to center)

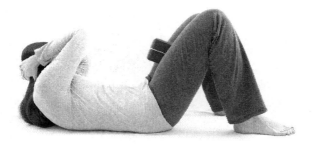

Bent Leg Twisting Abs with Block (exhale, twist to the left)

INSTRUCTION

- Lie flat on your back with knees bent and feet hips width apart. Feel free to use a blanket support (long rectangle fold) under the head.
- Place a yoga block (the middle thickness) between the thighs.
- Interlace hands behind the head, drawing the elbows in close together.
- Inhale, lift head and shoulders off the earth.
- Exhale, twist, pointing both elbows toward the right knee.
- Lift the left shoulder blade off the earth as you pull the navel down to the spine.
- Inhale, back to center, keeping head and shoulders off the earth.
- Exhale, twist, pointing elbows to the left knee.

- Inhale to center and continue.
- Repeat for 10 rounds (twisting toward both sides is considered a round).
- To release: remove the block and rest the hands on the belly. Take 4-5 long belly breaths while resting the knees together.
- Practice 2 more rounds, pausing between rounds for belly breaths.

BICYCLE ABS

This pose provides gentle movement for the hips and legs while working the abdominals. It gently stretches and releases tension in the hips and low back while strengthening core and hip muscles.

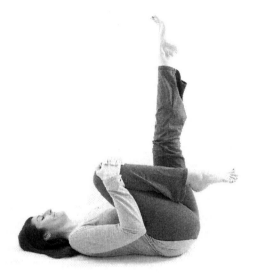

Bicycle Abs (inhale, lengthen leg toward sky)

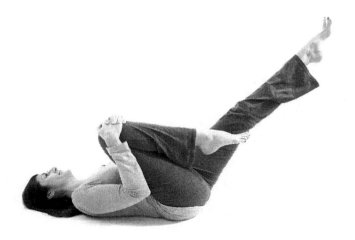

Bicycle Abs (exhale, slowly lower leg down)

YOGA FOR LOW BACK AND HIP HEALTH

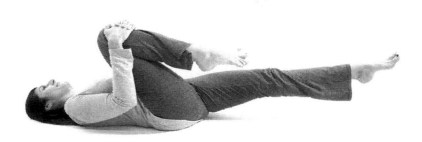

Bicycle Abs (exhale, slowly lower leg down and hover)

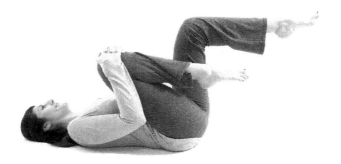

Bicycle Abs (inhale, hug knee back in and lengthen leg toward sky. Continue to repeat circular motion of the leg as though you were riding a bicycle)

INSTRUCTION

- Lie flat on your back with a blanket (long rectangle fold) under the head (option) and hug the right knee into the chest. Interlace the hands over or under the knee and soften the shoulders.
- Inhale, lengthen the left leg toward sky, reaching out through the toes. (Keep a bend in the knee if straightening the leg is too intense for the low back.)
- Exhale, slowly lower the left leg down so it hovers over the earth about an inch (if this feels like it's straining in the back, or feels like too much, hover the leg further away from the earth).

- Use your next inhale to bend the knee, hugging it back into the chest and lengthen it up toward sky.
- Exhale, slowly lower the leg down so it hovers.
- The extended leg is moving slowly, circling around, like riding a bicycle.
- Practice 10-20 rounds.
- Pause after the last round and rest the hands on the belly.
- Take 4-5 long belly breaths while resting the knees together.
- To transition to other side: hug left knee in and lengthen right leg toward sky. Follow same instruction.
- Practice 10-20 rounds.
- To release: rest the hands on the belly and take 4-5 long belly breaths while resting the knees together.
- Practice 2 more rounds on each side, pausing after each round for belly breaths.

PELVIC TILTS

This four part breath is designed to release the abs and stretch out tension in the low back area. It's great to practice after abdominal work and daily to stretch the low back and relieve pain. These are also helpful to strengthen a weak SI (sacroiliac) joint.

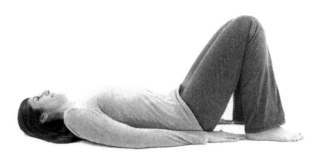

Pelvic Tilts Transiotion (open feet hip width, toes in line with heels, walk feet back to the buttocks so you can brush the fingertips to the heels)

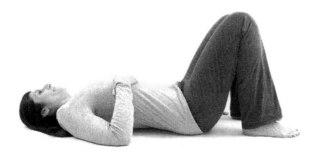

Pelvic Tilts (inhale, arch the low back, tailbone down, so there is a space between the back and earth)

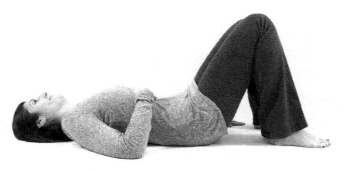

Pelvic Tilts (exhale, press low back into the earth)

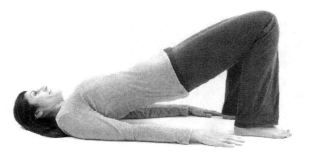

Pelvic Tilts (inhale, lift hips off the earth)

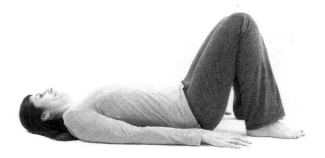

Pelvic Tilts (exhale, lower hips back down)

INSTRUCTION
- Lie flat on your back with knees bent and feet hips width

apart, with toes pointing forward in line with the heels, with no support under the head.
- Walk the feet back toward the buttocks and brush the heels with the fingertips.
- Inhale, arch the low back, drawing the tailbone down to the earth, keeping the hips on the earth (there will be a space between the low back and the earth).
- Exhale, press the low back into the earth, drawing the tailbone up toward the sky, pulling the navel down to the spine (low back is flat and hips are on the earth).
- Keeping the length in the low back, inhale, ground feet down and lift the hips up off the earth.
- Exhale, lower the hips back down.
- Inhale, arch low back.
- Exhale, press low back into the earth.
- Inhale, lift hips.
- Exhale, lower hips.
- Repeat and practice for 10-20 rounds.
- To release: hug the knees into the chest and breathe deeply for 5-10 slow breaths.

PLANK POSE

This pose is the ultimate core strengthening pose. A powerful way to connect to core muscles, build up heat and tone the arms and legs. When you practice Plank Pose, you are using the weight of the body to strengthen the core. This pose can be practiced with knees down for less intensity or legs straight for more. Be mindful of lifting out of the shoulders to prevent injury in the rotator cuff.

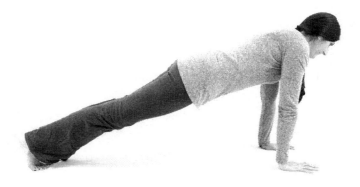

Plank Pose (straight legs)

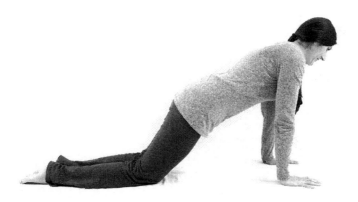

Plank Pose (knees down)

INSTRUCTION

- Starting on hands and knees, stack the wrists under the shoulders and spread the fingers wide.
- Gaze down with a long neck and spine as you step one leg back at a time, tucking the toes under. Feet can be close to together or hips width.
- Lift up through the shoulders and rock the weight forward, so wrists are under shoulders.
- Hips are parallel with the earth as you rock the weight forward.
- Soften the jaw and buttocks as you lift the navel to the spine.
- If straight legs are too intense, gently bring the knees down to the earth and continue to rock the weight forward engaging the core.
- Hold for 5-20 breaths (build up to a longer hold as you continue to practice. Bring the knees down to the earth as many times as you need, as you are building strength).
- To release: bring knees down if they aren't already and come into Child's Pose for 5-10 slow breaths (knees together for a low back stretch, knees apart for a hip stretch).
- Come back into Table Pose and hold Plank Pose for 2 more rounds pausing between each round in Child's Pose.

TABLE EXTENSIONS

Practiced on hands and knees, this pose strengthens the core, challenges balance and stretches the spine, arms and legs. It's the perfect pose to practice lifting out of the shoulders while making controlled movements from the center of the body.

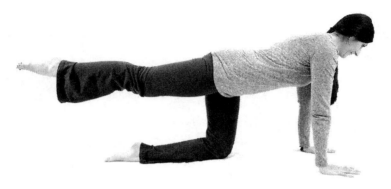

Table Extensions (right leg lengthened)

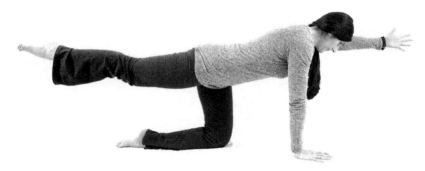

Table Extensions (right leg lengthened, left arm extended)

INSTRUCTION

- Come into Table Pose, stacking knees under hips and wrists under shoulders.
- With a neutral spine, inhale and extend right leg straight back, reaching through the toes, keeping the hip level. Toes off the earth.
- Exhale, draw navel to spine.

- For more intensity, inhale, lengthen left arm out, thumb toward sky.
- As you breathe, reach out through the fingers and toes and continue to draw the navel to the spine. Be sure to not sink into the low back.
- Lift out of the shoulders and be sure the right hip is not lifting up. You want length in the back leg, not height. Leg is level with the hip.
- There is a long line from the fingers to the toes and you pull the navel up and in, maintaining a straight spine with the gaze down. Neck is an extension of the spine.
- Hold for 10-20 breaths (build up to a longer hold as you continue to practice).
- To transition to other side: inhale, bring hand down. Exhale knee down. Come into Table Pose.
- Take 2 rounds of Cat/Cow Tilts.
- Come back to a neutral spine and switch sides. Repeat instructions for the left side.
- Practice up to 2 more rounds on each side again.
- To release: come back into Child's Pose for 10 slow cycles of breath.

CYNDI ROBERTS

CHAPTER TWO

RESTORATIVE YOGA POSE INSTRUCTION

BELLY DOWN ½ FROG

This supportive stretch softens and rests the muscles in the back of the hips and buttocks. With these muscles at rest, the pressure is taken off the sciatic nerve. Piriformis syndrome and sciatic nerve pain down the leg are thereby relieved.

While practicing this pose, the first chakra—the root chakra—is opened. The ability to ground is increased, thereby banishing fear in the body. Feeling comfortable in the body, feeling worthy of prosperity, and feeling safe and secure enough to let go and relax are developed as this energy balances.

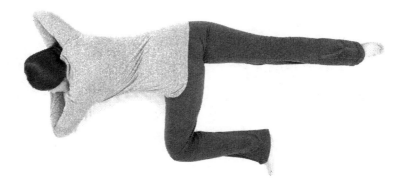

Belly Down ½ Frog (right leg bent at a 90 degree angle, head turned toward bent knee)

INSTRUCTION

- Starting in Table Pose, slowly lie down on your stomach.
- Bend the right knee and bring it in line with the hip (the leg will be at a right angle).
- Stack the forearms and rest the head down, turned toward the right.
- Close the eyes and breathe for 2-4 minutes.
- Transition to the other side: slowly straighten the bent leg, turn the head to the other side.

- Bend the left knee, bringing it in line with the hip, at a 90-degree angle.
- To release: straighten the bent leg and slowly come back into Table Pose and practice Child's Pose. Transition slowly and mindfully.

RECLINED ½ CRESCENT

This side opening position creates space in the hip, intercostal muscles of the ribs and top shoulder. As the side of the hip opens, tension in the pelvis dissolves, the hip flexors are gently stretched and breathing muscles soften. Deeper breaths create ease in the muscles and the mind.

While practicing this pose, the second chakra—the sacral chakra—and the third chakra—the solar plexus—are awakened, and emotional intelligence has the space to grow. The abilities to create healthy boundaries and gracefully move with the flow of life, without resistance to change, are enhanced. The energies of the right to act as your true self, connection to self-confidence and personal power with balanced self-esteem and ego-strength are boosted.

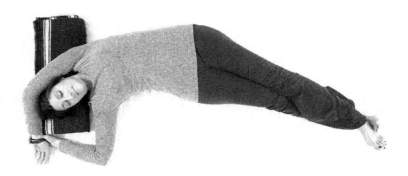

Reclined ½ Crescent (bending to the right, opening the left side)

INSTRUCTION

- Lie flat on the back with a blanket (long rectangle fold) under the head and the legs lengthened.
- Draw both legs over to the right side. Cross the left ankle over the right ankle.
- Inhale and stretch the arms overhead (the arms can rest by your sides if drawing them overhead isn't accessible). Bring

the arms and shoulders over to the right, creating a crescent shape with the body. For more stretch, grab onto the left wrist and gently tug. Release the wrist after a few breaths and allow the arms to rest naturally on the earth.
- Feel free to cover up with a blanket, place a blanket on the belly (large rectangle fold) for weight or use an eye pillow.
- Close the eyes and breathe slowly. Visualize the breath cascading through the side body, from fingers to toes.
- Hold each side for 3-5 minutes.
- To transition to the other side: uncross the ankles and bring the legs back to center. Bring the arms and shoulders back to center and take a full body stretch, reaching from fingertips to toes. Follow same instruction for the left side.
- To release: uncross the ankles and bring the legs back to center. Bring the arms and shoulders back to center and pause for a full body stretch. Option: hug the knees into the chest, place the hands on top of each knee and circle the knees in the same direction. Come onto your most comfortable side and take a few deep breaths before transitioning.

RECLINED LEG REST

In this position, the muscles in the abdomen, including the psoas, are able to rest. This restful state allows muscle contraction to release and utilizes gravity to bring the pelvis back into a neutral alignment. In this posture, tension in the low back melts away.

While practicing this position, the third chakra—the solar plexus chakra—energies are encouraged to open. The energies of the right to act as your true self, connection to self-confidence and personal power with balanced self-esteem and ego-strength are boosted. Having a balanced solar plexus chakra means you are connected to your true purpose in life. Living a life from the power emanating within renews your sense of joy for being alive and having purpose.

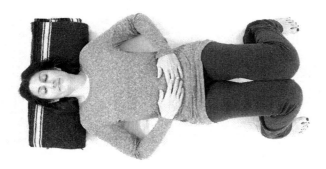

Reclined Leg Rest

INSTRUCTION
- Lie flat on the back with a blanket (long rectangle fold) under the head.
- Hug both knees into the chest and breathe for 5 deep breaths. Lengthen the tailbone and press the low back into the earth.
- On exhale, release the knees, resting the feet flat on the earth with bent knees, feet open wider than hips width, toes in line with heels, knees resting together.

- Hands can rest on the belly or by the sides. Feel free to cover up with a blanket, place a blanket on the belly (large rectangle fold) for weight or use an eye pillow.
- Close the eyes and connect to the image of the thighbones settling into the hip sockets. Imagine the muscles loosening as the weight of the legs melt down.
- Breathe deeply into the belly, hips and low back for 5-10 minutes.
- To release: open the knees up and practice Reclined Knee Hug (both knees). Hold for 4-5 cycles of breath and then circle the knees around in the same direction, releasing any remaining tension in the low back. Pause and switch directions of the circles and then come to stillness, hugging both knees in once more. Roll to one side and take a few deep breaths before coming up to seated. Transition slowly and mindfully.

SUPPORTED BELLY DOWN TWIST

This supported twist is extremely gentle and creates space to melt away tension and stress, not only in the mid-section but also the mind. All twists have a detoxing quality and support letting go in body and mind, especially when practiced for a long hold.

As the muscles of the torso soften, the muscles responsible for breathing soften, deepening the relaxation response in the body. Stress, anxiety, worries and concerns melt away with this self-soothing forward fold.

This calming posture stretches and relieves tension in the back and hips while resolving digestion issues and increasing lymphatic flow. Energy levels are boosted, and digestion and kidney function are stimulated.

While practicing this pose, the third chakra—the solar plexus—is ignited. The energies of the right to act as your true self, connection to self-confidence and personal power with balanced self-esteem and ego-strength are boosted. Having a balanced solar plexus means being connected to your true purpose in life. Living a life from the power emanating within naturally renews your sense of joy for being alive and having purpose.

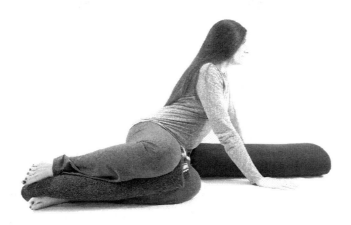

Supported Belly Down Twist Transition (hands frame the bolster, inhale, lengthen ribs – blanket, long rectangle fold, between knees and ankles)

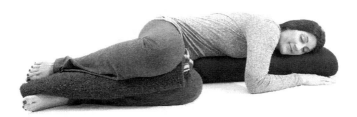

Supported Belly Down Twist (exhale, fold down – blanket, long rectangle fold, between knees and ankles)

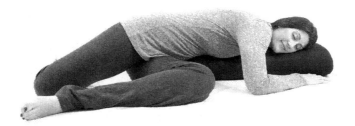

Supported Belly Down Twist (exhale, fold down – knees apart)

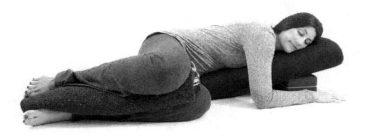

Supported Belly Down Twist (exhale, fold down – bolster propped on yoga block, blanket, long rectangle fold, between knees and ankles)

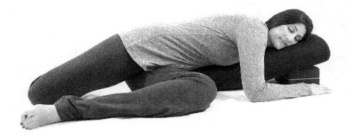

Supported Belly Down Twist (exhale, fold down – bolster propped on yoga block, knees apart)

INSTRUCTION

- Place a bolster vertically on the earth and have a few blankets and a yoga block nearby. Sit with one hip against a bolster. Stack the knees on top of each other to start, as you turn and face the bolster. Rest the hands on the earth on either side of the bolster.
- Inhale, lengthen the spine, drawing the ribs out of the waist.
- Exhale, fold down onto the bolster, resting the chest, torso and head down, facing the knees. If there is too much stretch, come up and place one or more folded blankets (long rectangle fold) on the bolster or prop the bolster on an angle with a yoga block.
- Soften the shoulders and take a deep breath. Which each breath out, allow the weight of the body to melt into the supports.

- Keep the knees together with a blanket (long rectangle fold) between knees and ankles or for more stretch in the hips, draw the top leg back, separating the knees. Option: place a folded blanket (large rectangle fold) on the top hip for weight.
- If you feel like you are falling off to one side, come up and readjust the bolster so it is directly in line with the hip.
- Breathe deeply for 5-7 minutes on each side. Imagine with each exhale that you are releasing tension in the spine, low back and hips. Cascade the breath the length of the spine, from crown to tailbone.
- If you would like to practice a mantra (words or phrase to focus the mind), silently repeat the words "let go." If you would like to match it to your breath, silently repeat "let" on inhale and "go" on exhale.
- To transition to other side: release the mantra if you were practicing it and slowly bring the knees together if the legs were wide. Press the hands into the earth to lift the torso up and turn away from the support. Continue to turn away, finding a comfortable seated position. Close the eyes and breathe for 2 slow cycles of breath, resetting the spine to neutral before you transition to the other side.
- Slowly open the eyes and continue to turn, bringing the left hip against the supports. Follow the same instruction for the other side.
- To release: bring the knees together, if wide, press the hands down to lift the torso up. Turn away from the supports and sit in a comfortable seat, taking a few slow breaths before transitioning.

SUPPORTED BELLY DOWN TWIST (EXTENDED LEG VARIATION)

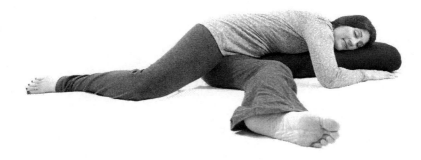

Supported Belly Down Twist (Extended Leg Variation)

INSTRUCTION

- Come into Supported Belly Down Twist.
- Slowly lengthen both legs, keeping a slight bend in the knees. For less intensity, bring the feet closer together. For more intensity, draw the feet further apart. Option: place a folded blanket (large rectangle fold) on the top hip for weight.
- Soften the shoulders and take a deep breath. Which each breath out, allow the weight of the body to melt into the support.
- Breathe deeply for 5-7 minutes on each side. Imagine, with each exhale, that you are releasing tension in the spine, side body and hips.
- Feel free to use the mantra as you practice this twist, silently repeat the words "let go." If you would like to match it to your breath, silently repeat "let" on inhale and "go" on exhale.
- To transition to other side: release the mantra if you were practicing it and slowly bring the knees together if the legs were wide. Press the hands into the earth to lift the torso up

and turn away from the support. Continue to turn away, finding a comfortable seated position. Close the eyes and breathe for 2 slow cycles of breath, resetting the spine to neutral before you transition to the other side. Slowly open the eyes and continue to turn, bringing the left hip against the supports. Follow the same instruction for the other side.

- To release: bring the knees together, if wide, press the hands down to lift the torso up. Turn away from the supports and sit in a comfortable seat, taking a few slow breaths before transitioning.

SUPPORTED BRIDGE WITH BENT LEGS

This pose counters tension in the low back, especially from sitting all day. It's beneficial for strengthening the SI (sacroiliac) joint and relieving tension in the sacrum. The pose allows the lower region of the lungs to open, thereby allowing space for deep breaths and release of stagnant air in the lungs. This opening of the ribs and chest also benefits the lungs, stimulating relaxation, thymus gland and immune function.

While practicing this pose, the fourth chakra—the heart chakra—and the fifth chakra—the throat chakra—are energized. Feeling worthy of being loved, loving unconditionally, immune function and ability to form healthy relationships are strengthened as the heart center opens.

Communication skills, speaking one's truth, creative expression and the ability to be a present listener are traits that are enhanced as the energies in the throat chakra are balanced.

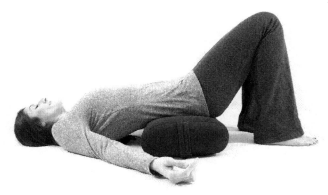

Supported Bridge with Bent Legs (bolster under low back, no support under head)

INSTRUCTION

- Place a bolster by your side and lie flat on the earth with no support under the head.

YOGA FOR LOW BACK AND HIP HEALTH

- Bend the knees and rest the feet flat on the earth, hips width apart, toes and heels in a line. Walk the heels back close to the buttocks so ankles are stacked under the knees.
- Ground the feet down and lift the hips up on inhale. Slide the bolster under the low back/sacrum area and lower the hips back down, resting the low back/sacrum on the bolster. Be sure that the bolster is in a place where you feel supported, making adjustments as needed.
- If using the bolster is too much stretch, use a blanket (long rectangle fold) under the sacrum/low back.
- Keep grounding the feet into the earth as you allow the hips and low back to completely rest on the support.
- Walk the tips of the shoulder blades close together and then let them rest naturally.
- Open the arms out like wings or rest the arms by your sides. You can even rest the arms overhead for more stretch in the shoulders and lymph glands.
- Feel free to cover up with a blanket, place a blanket on the belly (large rectangle fold) or use an eye pillow.
- Breathe deeply into the belly, ribs and chest for 3-5 minutes.
- To release: ground the feet down and gently lift the hips up to slide the bolster or blanket out. Lengthen the tailbone and slowly lower the hips back down and practice Reclined Knee Hug (both knees) to reset the spine and release the low back. Option: bring the hands on top of each knee and circle the knees around in the same direction.

SUPPORTED CHILD'S POSE

The ultimate restorative yoga posture for safety, letting go, comfort and relaxation. This pose creates flexibility in the back, hips and knees as you breathe deeply in a nurtured and supported space.

Practicing Supported Child's Pose gently stretches hip and back muscles, while the breath gently massages the abdominal organs. The nervous system calms, turns the relaxation response on, combats anxiety and stress, improves digestion, lowers blood pressure, and relieves insomnia.

While practicing this pose, all seven chakra energies open, from root to crown. Supported Child's Pose is particularly beneficial for the three lower chakra energies: root, sacral and solar plexus. This pose is a grounding position, reaffirming your right to be here, your right to feel and the right to be your true self.

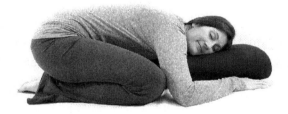

Supported Child's Pose

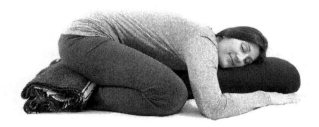

Supported Child's Pose (blanket, long rectangle fold, on heels)

INSTRUCTION

- Start in Table Pose, place a bolster vertically on the earth in front of you (have a few extra blankets nearby in case you need them).
- Open the knees out to the edges of the bolster and bring the big toes together. Sit back on the heels. For more stretch in the hips, open the knees wider than the bolster.
- Draw the bolster back between the knees and lay the chest and torso down on the bolster.
- Be sure the chest is level with the hips and stack up as many folded blankets (long rectangle fold) on the bolster as you need to. If there is any pain in the knees, place a blanket (long rectangle fold) on the heels and sit back.
- Turn the head to one side for 3 to 4 minutes. Then turn the head to the other side for 3 to 4 minutes. Your total time in the pose will be 6-8 minutes.
- If turning the head isn't accessible, place a blanket (square fold) or block on the bolster and rest the forehead on it.
- Close the eyes, soften the belly and imagine that you can inhale through the crown of the head, all the way down the spine, to the back of the hips and low back. Exhale out from the hips, up the spine, out through the crown, releasing any tension or holding.
- To release: come onto hands and knees into Table Pose and stretch one leg back at a time, opening up the back of the leg, practicing Modified Downward Facing Dog or come into Downward Facing Dog and "walk the dog", until the compression in the back of the legs is released. Transition slowly and mindfully.

SUPPORTED FINAL RELAXATION

This supported position is extremely gentle, accessible for most and takes the pressure off the low back. Added support creates a deeper, safer space for letting go so you can allow the body to drift into relaxation and well-being.

As the entire body is able to relax, energy reserves are directed toward healing, organs rest and the nervous system calms. This calming posture is ideal for deep states of relaxation, meditation, healing and practicing yoga nidra.

While practicing this pose, all energies of the chakra system flow freely, uniting the rainbow energies through breath and relaxation. Physical and emotional energies are balanced with the egoic self. Social identity, creativity, self-identity and universal connection unite as relaxation and homeostasis are achieved.

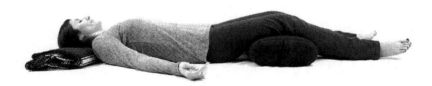

Supported Final Relaxation (arms out)

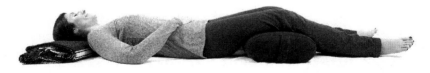

Supported Final Relaxation (hands on belly)

YOGA FOR LOW BACK AND HIP HEALTH

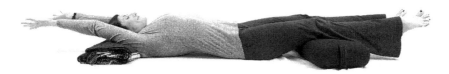

Supported Final Relaxation Transition (full body stretch)

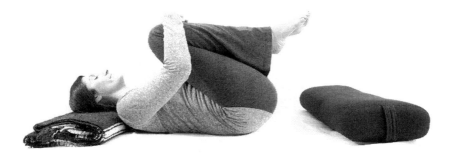

Supported Final Relaxation Transition (Reclined Knee Hug, both knees)

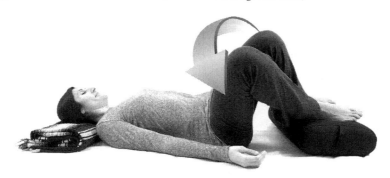

Supported Final Relaxation Transition (bend legs, rock knees side to side)

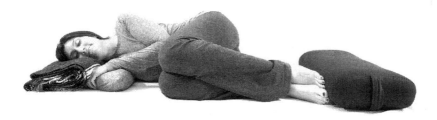

Supported Final Relaxation Transition (lay on most comfortable side)

INSTRUCTION

- Lie flat on the back and use a blanket (long rectangle fold) under the head and a bolster under the backs of the knees.
- Lengthen the legs out over the bolster, rest the heels on the earth and allow the legs and feet to relax.
- Rest the hands on the belly, bring the arms out to the side or open the arms out wide. Feel free to cover up with a blanket, place a blanket on the belly (large rectangle fold) or use an eye pillow.
- Close the eyes and take slow, full breaths, dropping into relaxation, melting away stress. Allow the body to melt into the earth and supports beneath you.
- Hold for 5-8 minutes.
- If you would like to practice a mantra (words or a phrase to focus the mind), as you inhale, silently repeat "inhale," as you exhale, silently repeat "exhale."
- In traditional yoga classes, the awareness is encouraged to drift and the breath is encouraged to become natural as the student practices Final Relaxation. I invite students to practice deep breaths and mantras to keep the focus inward and receive more benefits from the practice.
- To release: take a deep breath and make small movements; wiggle fingers and toes or circle wrists and ankles. Lengthen the arms overhead and take a full body stretch, stretching from fingers to toes. Exhale, practice Reclined Knee Hug (both knees) or bend the legs and rock the knees side to side.
- Roll onto your most comfortable side and pause several deep breaths to reset before transitioning.

SUPPORTED ½ MOON

This restorative side opening position creates space in the hips, low back, intercostal muscles of the ribs and shoulders. The pelvis naturally realigns while tension is eased in the low back. Tension in the side body restricting the diaphragm is cleared, so breathing becomes easier.

Lungs are strengthened and the relaxation response is more accessible with deeper breaths. This is an ideal pose to open the side body before coming into deep twists. Finding length before coming into a twist protects the spine and low back. This variation of the pose is extremely gentle on the shoulders, but still provides an adequate stretch for the top shoulder.

While practicing this pose, the second chakra—the sacral chakra—and the third chakra—the solar plexus—are awakened. Emotional intelligence has the space to grow as you are more able to create healthy boundaries. The ability to gracefully move with the flow of life, without resistance to change, is enhanced. The energies of the right to act as your true self, connection to self-confidence and personal power with balanced self-esteem and ego-strength are boosted as both of these chakras come into alignment.

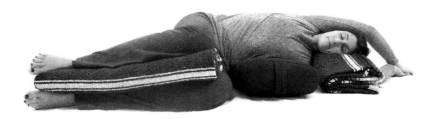

Supported ½ Moon (bottom arm lenghtened with top arm overhead. Blankets, long rectangle fold, between knees and ankles and on top of bottom shoulder)

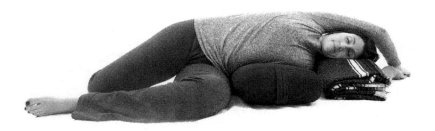

Supported ½ Moon (bottom arm lenghtened with top arm overhead, blanket, long rectangle fold, on top of bottom shoulder. Knees apart)

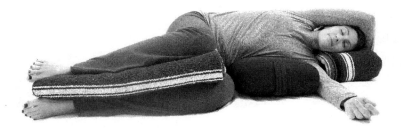

Supported ½ Moon (straight bottom arm with top arm overhead. Blanket, long rectangle fold, between knees and ankles)

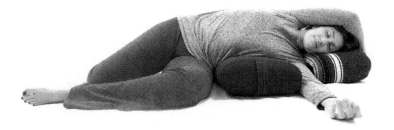

Supported ½ Moon (straight bottom arm with top arm overhead. Knees apart)

YOGA FOR LOW BACK AND HIP HEALTH

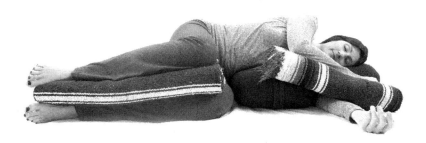

Supported ½ Moon (straight bottom arm, top arm rests on blanket, small rectangle fold. Blanket, long rectangle fold, between knees and ankles)

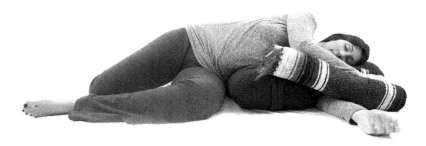

Supported ½ Moon (straight bottom arm, top arm rests on blanket, small rectangle fold. Knees apart)

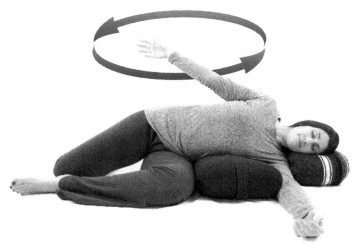

Supported ½ Moon (arm circles, straight arm)

INSTRUCTION

- Place your bolster horizontally on the earth. Sit with the right hip up against the bolster.
- There are two variations for the bottom shoulder – for most stretch – use an inhale to lengthen the ribs and as you exhale, drape the rib cage on the bolster as you lengthen the bottom arm, palm up, resting it on the earth. Place a blanket (long rectangle fold) on the bottom shoulder and rest the head on.
- Stack the knees on top of each with a blanket (long rectangle fold) between the knees and ankles or stagger the legs, scissoring the top leg back for more stretch.
- Legs can stay bent or straighten. If your leg or legs are straight, be sure to keep a slight bend in the knee to protect the knee from hyperextension.
- Inhale top arm up and over the head. Gently tug the top wrist to get a little more stretch on inhale. As you exhale, release the wrist and allow the hands to softly rest on the earth.
- If this is too much stretch for the top shoulder, rest the arm out in front of you under a blanket (small rectangle fold). Option: place a folded blanket (large rectangle fold) on the top hip for weight.
- For less stretch in the bottom shoulder – place a blanket (square fold) on the earth to use as a support under the head – about 12 inches away from the bolster.
- Inhale, lengthen the ribs and as you exhale, drape the rib cage on the bolster. Head rests on the blanket, bottom arm lengthens out on the earth in front of you, palm up toward sky.
- Stack the knees on top of each with a blanket (long rectangle fold) between the knees and ankles or stagger the legs, scissoring the top leg back for more stretch.

- Legs can stay bent or straighten. If your leg or legs are straight, be sure to keep a slight bend in the knee to protect the knee from hyperextension.
- Use an inhale to lengthen the top arm over the head. Rest the hand palm down (if this is too much stretch for the top shoulder, rest the arm out in front of you under a blanket, small rectangle fold). Option: place a folded blanket (large rectangle fold) on the top hip for weight.
- Close the eyes and drop right into deep breaths. Breathe into the places you feel the stretch and expansion of the side body. When the awareness drifts, keep coming back to the breath and feeling what is there for you in the moment. Allow yourself to feel but also allow for the breath to melt away tension and holding.
- Option: Arm Circles – before you transition out of the pose, take a few minutes to practice some gentle yoga for the top arm. Inhale, lengthen the top arm toward sky and as you exhale, slowly circle the arm around. If circling a straight arm isn't accessible, bend the arm and circle the elbow. These circles gently stretch the top shoulder and loosen tension in the shoulder joint. Slower circles are more beneficial. Practice with deep breaths for 10-20 cycles of breath.
- To transition to the other side: draw the knees together if they were apart or bend the legs if they were straight. Press the top hand into the bolster and come up to seated. Turn slowly away from the bolster and pause in a comfortable seated position. Close the eyes and breathe for 2 slow cycles of breath, resetting the spine to neutral before you transition to the other side. Slowly open the eyes and continue to turn, bringing the left hip against the supports. Follow the same instruction for the other side.

- To release: draw the knees together if they were apart or bend the legs if they were straight. Press the top hand into the bolster and come up to seated. Turn to face away from the support and find a comfortable seated position. Take a few deep breaths before transitioning.

SUPPORTED INVERSION

This safe and gentle supported inversion allows for a change in perspective as you turn your world upside down. Reverse gravity as you allow the organs to rest, shift lymphatic flow, bring fresh blood back to the heart and brain, improve immune function, foster mental clarity and give the legs and feet a much needed rest. Practice to relieve stress from a long day or counter jet lag after a long flight.

While practicing this supported inversion, you are increasing the energy flow of the upper chakra centers. The fifth chakra—the throat chakra, the sixth chakra—the third eye center—and the seventh chakra—the crown chakra—energies open.

Enhance truthful communication, creative expression and establish the basic rights to speak and be heard as the throat chakra clears. Establish personal identity, develop intuition and the ability to think symbolically as the energies in the third eye center open. Stagnant energies in the crown chakra are released as connections to wisdom, spirituality, higher understanding and the basic rights to know and learn are made while practicing this posture.

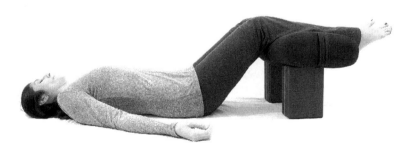

Supported Inversion (arms out)

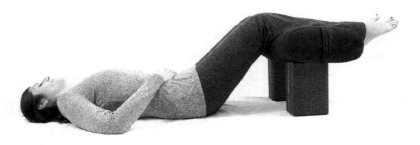

Supported Inversion (hands on belly)

INSTRUCTION

- Place 2 blocks on the highest setting, on the earth about 12 inches apart. Place a bolster horizontally on top of the blocks.
- Facing the supports, slowly, one leg at a time, drape the legs over the support, resting the backs of the calf muscles on top of the bolster. Slowly and mindfully, lie down on the earth.
- Head and shoulders rest flat on the earth, with no support under the head.
- Rest hands on belly or arms by the sides. Turn your palms up for more of an opening in the chest. You can also bring the arms out to a "T," bringing wrists and shoulders in a line. Feel free to cover up with a blanket, place a blanket on the belly (large rectangle fold) or use an eye pillow.
- Close the eyes and breathe slowly for 8-10 minutes.
- Allow the muscles to soften as any tension or stress flows down and out through the crown of the head. The mind clears as the body lets go.
- To release: inhale and take a full body stretch, reaching from fingertips to toes. On exhale, hug the knees into the chest. Take a few deep breaths in stillness, pressing the low back into the earth. You can also bring the hands on each knee and circle the knees in the same direction to release any remaining tension in the low back.

- Slowly roll to one side and rest for a few moments, resetting the spine before you come up to seated. Transition slowly.

SIDE LYING POSE

Side lying pose is accessible to everyone and is especially useful for those looking to reduce stress, lower blood pressure, relieve fatigue and help soothe digestion upset. It's an ideal pose for rest, meditation, yoga nidra, sleep, and the ultimate pose of comfort and self-soothing.

While practicing this pose, all of the chakras come into alignment. The energies of all the chakra centers move across the rainbow bridge, finding balance with each deep breath.

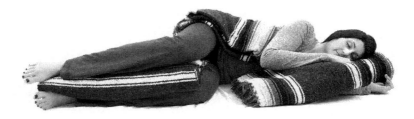

Side Lying Pose (blanket, square fold, under the head, blanket, small rectangle fold, under top arm, blanket, long rectangle fold, between knees and ankles and blanket, large rectangle fold on hip)

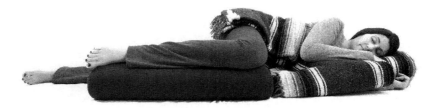

Side Lying Pose (blanket, square fold, under the head, blanket, small rectangle fold, under top arm, blanket, large rectangle fold on hip and straight bottom leg with bent top leg resting on bolster)

INSTRUCTION

- Gently and slowly, come down on to the earth and rest on your most comfortable side. Place a folded blanket (square fold) under the head. Place another blanket (long rectangular

- fold) between the knees and ankles or straighten bottom leg, bend top leg and rest it on a bolster.
- Hug one or two folded blankets (small rectangle fold), like you're hugging a teddy bear. This helps soften and reduce and stress on the top shoulder. It also provides additional comfort and support.
- For more support and comfort, place a folded blanket (large rectangle fold) on the top hip and low back or lean up the back up against the wall. Feel free to cover up with another blanket.
- Slightly shift the bottom hip back and roll the top hip forward so the hip joints are not stacked on top of each other. Move the bottom shoulder back slightly as the top shoulder rolls slightly forward.
- Soften the belly and breathe deep and slow. Feel the breath in the body as you witness each inhale and exhale with a gentle awareness.
- Hold for 10-15 minutes. Imagine the body resting in comfort, ease and safety.
- If you would like to focus the mind, practice a loving kindness meditation by silently repeating, "May I be peaceful and at ease. May I be happy and healthy." Each time the awareness wanders, compassionately bring it back to silently repeating the meditation.
- To release: move the props away and gently press up into a comfortable seat. Transition slowly.

SUPPORTED PIGEON POSE

This supported hip opener is ideal to relieve built-up tension in the hips from sitting for long periods of time. Most of us, especially women, store emotions in the hips. When we stretch this area with a longer hold, we essentially clear out stagnation in this emotional storehouse, releasing what we are ready to be free of.

This is a powerful pose that opens the hips and backs of the legs. It relieves tension in the low back, tightness in the piriformis muscle and eases sciatic nerve pain. It's ideal to counter pain from piriformis syndrome.

While practicing this pose, the energies of the first chakra—the root chakra—and the second chakra—the sacral chakra—are cleared. Connection to health, vitality, feelings of safety, establishing trust in the world, finding stability and manifesting prosperity are restored as you open the root chakra energy.

Emotional intelligence is enhanced. Healthy boundaries can be established, enjoying pleasure in a healthy manner and not resisting change are characteristics that are nurtured as the sacral energies flow freely.

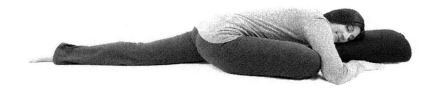

Supported Pigeon Pose (right leg forward, torso resting on bolster)

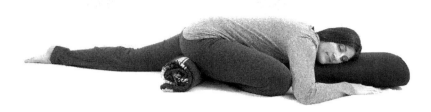

Supported Pigeon Pose (right leg forward, torso resting on bolster with blanket roll under the hips)

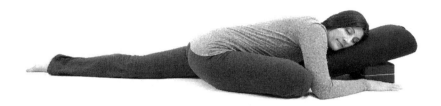

Supported Pigeon Pose (right leg forward, torso resting on bolster propped on yoga block)

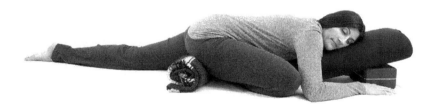

Supported Pigeon Pose (right leg forward, torso resting on bolster propped on yoga block and blanket roll under the hips)

INSTRUCTION

- Starting in Table Pose, place a bolster vertically out in front of you (have extra blankets and a block nearby).
- Draw the right knee to the right wrist and pivot the right foot over to the left as you lengthen the left leg straight back.
- Stay on hands as you center the hips and rest the top of the back foot down on the earth. Hips are level.

- Right heel is close to the groin for less intensity, further away for more intensity.
- Place a blanket roll under both hips to help align hips and add support.
- This pose is a deep hip opener and may be intense. You do not want to be in pain or unable to relax into the stretch, so be honest with yourself about what feels like too much stretch. Also be aware of what is too little stretch. I encourage you to find your edge—the first place of resistance—and breathe there so the muscles release and you gain flexibility.
- Still on hands, take a breath in and lift the waist out of the hips. As you exhale, fold down, resting the torso down on the bolster and turn the head toward the bent knee. Rest the forearms and hands on the earth, softening the shoulders as you exhale.
- Let the bolster hold the weight of the upper body. Adjust the bolster and stack up as many folded blankets (long rectangular fold) or prop the bolster up with a block, as you need to be completely comfortable and able to let go.
- Breathe slowly for 4-7 minutes, depending on desired intensity, each side.
- To transition to the other side: slowly come to hands and knees into Table Pose. Practice Modified Downward Facing Dog, stretching one leg back at a time, or practice Downward Facing Dog and "walk the dog," releasing compression in the leg. Come back into Table Pose when you are ready and follow the same instruction for the left side.
- To release: slowly come back to hands and knees in Table Pose. Practice Modified Downward Facing Dog, stretching one leg back at a time or practicing Downward Facing Dog and "walk the dog," releasing compression in the leg. Transition slowly.

SUPPORTED RECLINING POSE

This favorite and extremely calming chest opening posture is helpful to reduce stress, stretch out tension in the neck, shoulders, chest and low back. This back bend boosts immune function and is helpful to relieve depression. It's also helpful to counteract insomnia, acid reflux and coughing.

While practicing this pose, the fourth chakra—the heart center—and the fifth chakra—the throat chakra—open and clear. As the heart chakra opens, heartache is relieved and the connection to love and compassion, for self and others is enhanced. Open energy of the throat chakra allows space to speak your truth and express your needs in a kind and honest way.

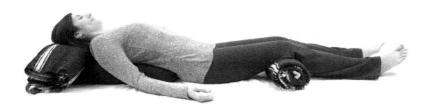

Supported Reclining Pose (back on bolster, blanket, long rectangle fold, behind head, blanket roll under knees)

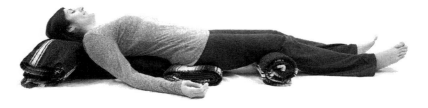

Supported Reclining Pose (back on bolster, blanket, long rectangle fold, behind head, blanket roll under knees with blanket, long rectangle fold, under buttocks)

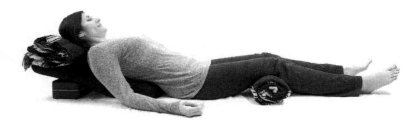

Supported Reclining Pose (back on bolster propped on a block, blanket, long rectangle fold, behind head, blanket roll under knees)

INSTRUCTION

- Place a bolster support vertically on the earth and a folded blanket (long rectangle fold) horizontally on the bolster where your head is going to be (have an extra blanket and yoga block nearby).
- Sit facing away from the bolster, with your low back against the edge of the bolster. If you have a very tight low back, place a folded blanket (long rectangle fold) horizontally on the earth against the bolster and sit on it.
- Place a blanket roll or another bolster under the knees.
- Lie back on the bolster and adjust the blanket under the head. You should feel a slight stretch in the low back, chest and shoulders when you lie back, but no sharp pain. Come out immediately and adjust if you're feeling pain. Try adding a blanket under the buttocks to sit on (long rectangle fold) if you haven't already or use another blanket if one isn't enough.
- Lengthen the legs out over the blanket roll so the heels rest on the earth. Lift the hips slightly and lengthen the low back and then rest the hips back down.
- Rest the arms by your side, either close to the torso, for less stretch in the chest and shoulders or further away for more

stretch. Roll the palms up toward sky for more opening in the shoulders or keep palms down for grounding.
- Feel free to cover up with a blanket, place a blanket on the belly (large rectangle fold) or use an eye pillow.
- Close the eyes and breathe deep into the belly, ribs and chest, opening the heart, while focusing on the breath. Keep coming back to feeling the stretch and breath when the focus drifts.
- Breathe deeply and slowly for 10-20 minutes. If you would like to practice a mantra (words or phrase to focus the mind), silently repeat, "I am light. I am love," allowing this positive affirmation to focus the mind and center the heart and throat chakras.
- To release: slowly bend the legs and gently roll onto the forearm of one side and then gently press up to seated. Close the eyes and take a few breaths, lifting the sternum as the spine resets to neutral. Transition slowly.

SUPPORTED RESTING BUTTERFLY

This forward fold is a pose of surrender and is therefore very calming to the nervous system. As your stress level lowers, the low back and hips gently stretch away tension and strengthen the energy flow of the legs. This pose is helpful to relieve menstrual cramps, lower blood pressure and insomnia. With each deep breath, the digestive organs are being gently massaged, stimulating digestion and improving abdominal organ function.

While practicing this pose, the first chakra—the root chakra—and the second chakra—the sacral chakra—are gently brought back into balance. The ability to ground is increased, thereby banishing fear in the body.

Feeling comfortable in the body, feeling worthy of prosperity and feeling safe and secure enough to let go and relax are developed as the root chakra energy balances. Emotional intelligence has the space to grow. The abilities to create healthy boundaries and gracefully move with the flow of life, without resistance to change, are enhanced. as the sacral chakra opens.

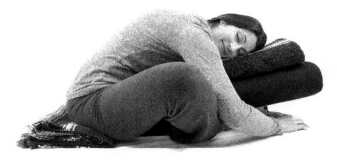

Supported Resting Butterfly (seated on blanket, long rectangle fold, resting torso on bolster and blanket, long rectangle fold)

YOGA FOR LOW BACK AND HIP HEALTH

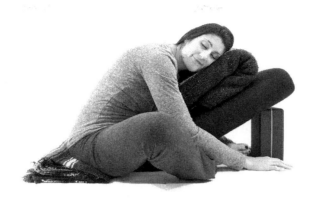

Supported Resting Butterfly (seated on blanket, long rectangle fold, resting torso on bolster propped on yoga block, head on blanket, square fold, turned to one side)

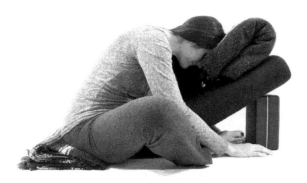

Supported Resting Butterfly (seated on blanket, long rectangle fold, resting torso on bolster propped on yoga block, forehead on blanket, square fold)

INSTRUCTION

- Sit on a folded blanket (long rectangular fold) with the soles of the feet together, knees open out. The legs will form a diamond shape. Draw the sit bones back and rock the pelvis forward.
- The closer the heels are to the groin, the more intense the stretch will be. I encourage you to take a wider butterfly, drawing the heels further away from the groin, because this is a long hold and intensity will build as you rest.

- Place your bolster vertically, stacked with blankets (long rectangle fold), resting on the legs and feet.
- If you need a higher support, place a block under the bolster, close to the toes. The other end of the bolster will rest between the legs on the earth. The bolster will be at an angle. Place a folded blanket (small square fold) on top of the bolster and rest the forehead down. You can also turn the head to one side. Be mindful of what feels better on the neck.
- Take an inhale and lift the ribs out of the waist and as you exhale, fold down onto the support.
- Let the shoulders melt down the back and make any adjustments you need before coming to stillness.
- Take slow and soft breaths. Imagine you can breathe in through the crown of the head down to the hips and exhale out from the hips into the earth. Release any tension and holding in the hips, slowly opening up the low back.
- Hold for 5-8 minutes. If the head is turned to one side, be sure to split the time equally between each direction the head is turned.
- To release: Bring torso back to center and clear props away. Hands come to the outside of the legs and gently draw the knees together as you straighten the legs. Bring the hands behind you and gently shake out the legs and circle the ankles.

CHAPTER THREE

GENTLE YOGA POSE INSTRUCTION

CAT/COW TILTS

Previously, I discussed how moving the spine in each of its six directions is helpful to release built up back tension. Cat/Cow Tilts move the spine in two directions, creating space between the discs from the tailbone through the neck. Cat Tilt is a slight forward fold, where the spine lengthens. Cow Tilt is a slight backbend, where the spine gently compresses.

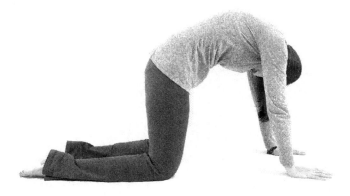

Cat Tilt (exhale, round back. Forward fold, spine lengthens)

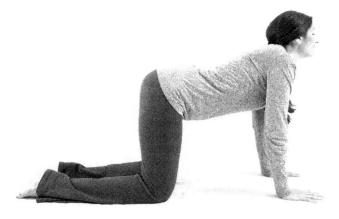

Cow Tilt (inhale, ribs forward. Back bend, spine compresses)

INSTRUCTION

- Come into Table Pose. If there is discomfort in the knees, place a blanket (large rectangle fold or long rectangle fold) under them for more padding.
- Start with a strong foundation by stacking the wrists under the shoulders and the knees under the hips.
- Inhale, drop the belly and arch the low back. Pull the ribs and chest forward and if it's okay for the neck, gaze up toward sky.
- As you exhale, round the back, press up through the back of the shoulder blades and gaze down or between the legs.
- Practice 10 – 15 rounds.
- To release: come to a neutral spine.

CHILD'S POSE

Practicing Child's Pose gently stretches hip and back muscles, while the breath gently massages the abdominal organs. It is a true resting pose and soothes the nervous system.

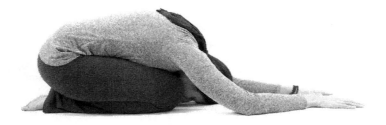

Child's Pose (knees together, forehead on the earth, arms lengthened out)

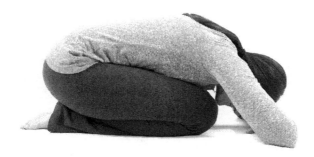

Child's Pose (knees together, forehead on forearms)

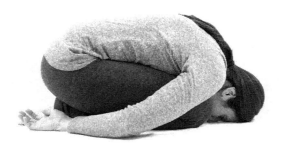

Child's Pose (knees together, forehead on the earth, arms by sides)

YOGA FOR LOW BACK AND HIP HEALTH

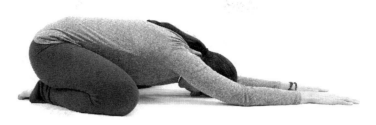

Child's Pose (knees wide, forehead on the earth, arms out)

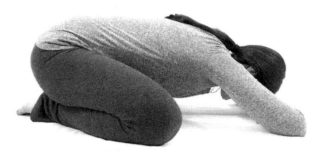

Child's Pose (knees wide, forehead on forearms)

INSTRUCTION

- If you would like to stretch the low back, start in Table Pose and keep the knees close together.
- Take a deep breath in and as you exhale, sit back on the heels. Rest the head on the earth or stack the forearms and rest the head on top.
- For more stretch in the shoulders, lengthen the arms out in front of you. For less stretch, stack the forearms on top of each other and rest the forehead down on the arms. You can also rest the forehead on a block or blanket (square fold) if the forehead doesn't reach the ground or arms. For no stretch in the shoulders, rest the arms by your side.
- If you would like to stretch the hips, start in Table Pose and open the knees out wide.
- Take a deep breath in and as you exhale, sit back on the heels. Rest the head on the earth or stack the forearms and rest the head on top.

- For more stretch in the shoulders, lengthen the arms out in front of you. For less stretch, stack the forearms on top of each other and rest the forehead down on the arms. You can also rest the forehead on a block or blanket (square fold) if the forehead doesn't reach the ground or arms. For no stretch in the shoulders, rest the arms by your side.
- Close the eyes, soften the belly and imagine that you can inhale through the crown of the head, all the way down the spine, to the back of the hips and low back. Exhale out from the hips, up the spine, out through the crown, releasing any tension or holding.
- To release: come back into Table Pose and stretch one leg back at a time, opening up the back of the leg, practicing Modified Downward Facing Dog or come into Downward Facing Dog and "walk the dog", until the compression in the back of the legs is released. Transition slowly and mindfully.

DOWNWARD FACING DOG

This pose incorporates a full body stretch and is a phenomenal way to stretch shoulders, hips, hamstrings and the backs of the legs. "Walking the dog" provides a deeper stretch to the backs of the legs and hamstrings, releasing compression and relieving muscle cramps or tension.

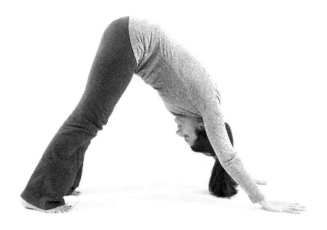

Downward Facing Dog

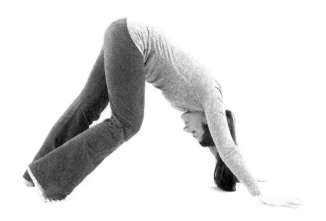

Downward Facing Dog (walking the dog, right leg bends as left leg lengthens)

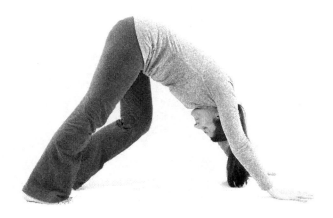

Downward Facing Dog (walking the dog, left leg bends as right leg lengthens)

INSTRUCTION

- Come onto hands and knees in Table Pose.
- Spread fingers wide and tuck the toes under.
- Lift the knees off the earth and draw the chest toward the thighs. Open feet hips width apart.
- Continue to draw the chest back to the thighs as you send the heels down to the earth with straight legs.
- If the shoulders are tight, open the hands wider than shoulder width. Spread and press the fingers into the earth and lift out of the shoulders.
- To "walk the dog," bend one leg as you lengthen the other, shifting back and forth between legs until the legs are stretched.
- Take as many rounds as you need to stretch the backs of the legs and feel free to pause for a few breaths in stillness, working the heels down to the earth as you draw the chest to the thighs.
- To release: bend the legs and gently place them down on the earth, coming back into Table Pose.

HIP CIRCLES

As you circle the leg around, the weight of the leg massages the muscles of the hip and low back, easing tension not only in the muscles but also in the ligaments and soft tissue. Moving the joint lubricates it, thereby improving flexibility and relieving aches and soreness in the hip and low back.

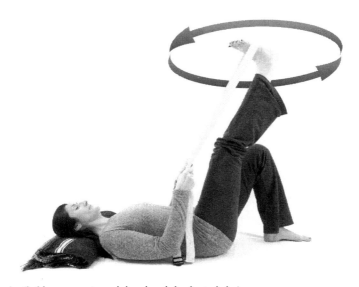

Hip Circles (hold one strap in each hand and slowly circle leg)

INSTRUCTION

- Place a strap next to you and lie flat on your back with a blanket (long rectangle fold) under the head.
- Bend the knees so both feet rest flat on the earth and draw the right knee into the chest. Place the strap around the foot and lengthen the leg toward the sky. Press out through the heel as you straighten the leg to the best of your ability.
- Hold one strap in each hand, and slowly circle the leg around.
- Left leg can stay bent for more support or you can lengthen it out and rest it on the earth.

- As you circle the leg, allow the leg to be passive. The work is coming from the arms while the shoulders and hands remain soft. Release the jaw if you are tightening it.
- Gently and slowly make large circles as you breathe deeply for 10-20 cycles of breath.
- To transition to the other side: bend the leg and remove the strap. Hug the left knee in and place the strap around the left leg. Follow same instructions for left side.
- To release: bend the leg and remove the strap.

LOW LUNGE HANDS ON THIGH

This powerful hip opener stretches both the front and back of the hips, releasing built up tension while taking pressure off the low back.

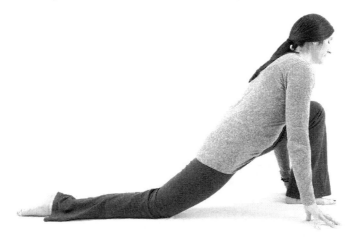

Low Lunge Hands on Thigh Transition (hands on the earth to come into the pose)

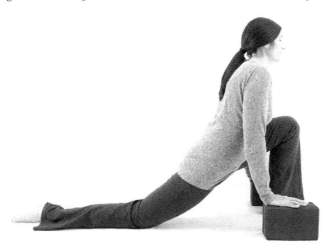

Low Lunge Hands on Thigh Transition (hands on blocks to come into the pose)

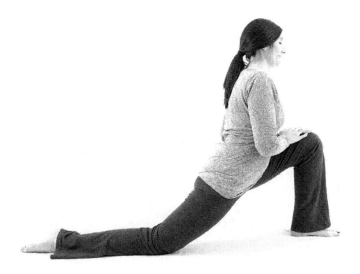

Low Lunge Hands on Thigh

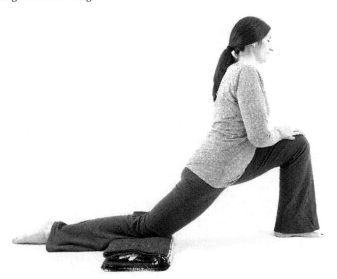

Low Lunge Hands on Thigh (blanket, long rectangle fold, under the back knee)

INSTRUCTION

- Come into Table Pose.
- Step the right foot between the hands and align the right knee over the right ankle. Use blocks under the hands if you need

assistance getting into the pose and use a blanket under the back knee if you need padding.
- Center the hips.
- Rest the top of the back foot down on the earth, engage the core and as you inhale, bring both hands onto the thigh.
- Soften the shoulders and keep a soft and steady gaze; this pose may challenge your balance.
- Keep drawing the hips forward without passing the right knee beyond the right ankle to protect the knee joint.
- For more stretch, come back down onto hands and draw the left knee back. Bring the hands back onto the knee.
- Soften the front toes and jaw as you breathe for 20-30 slow breaths.
- To transition to the other side: bring hands down and come back into Table Pose. Step left foot between the hands and follow instructions for the left side.
- To release: gently place the hands on the earth and step back into Table Pose.

MODIFIED DOWNWARD FACING DOG

This modified pose is accessible, easy on the shoulders and a gentle way to stretch the hips, hamstrings, calf muscles and Achilles tendons. It also provides release of compression in the leg, is useful to relieve cramps in the calf muscle and stretches the toes. It is a gentle way to stretch the back of the entire leg.

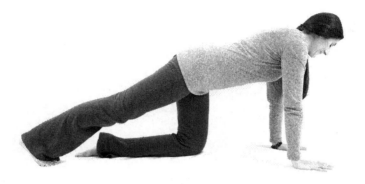

Modified Downward Facing Dog (right leg back)

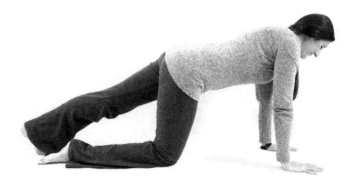

Modified Downward Facing Dog (left leg back)

INSTRUCTION

- Come into Table Pose.
- Stack wrists under shoulders and knees under hips. Use an inhale to stretch the right leg back keeping the toes on the earth.

- Tuck toes under and press out through the heel, opening up the back of the leg and releasing compression.
- Keep the arms straight without hyperextending into the elbows.
- Neck is long, gaze is down.
- To transition to other side: use an exhale to bring the right knee down under the hip. Inhale and lengthen the left leg back, tuck toes under and press out through the heel.
- Continue with the breath and switch the legs back and forth until the backs of the legs have been stretched open.

RECLINED KNEE DOWN TWIST

This twist is a way to unwind the spine while opening the chest, shoulder, arm and lymph glands. It's a gentle way to move out remaining compression or tension in the low back. It is also detoxing and deep breaths gently massage abdominal organs.

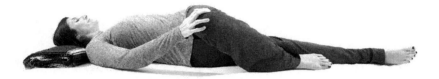

Reclined Knee Down Twist (left knee down, head neutral)

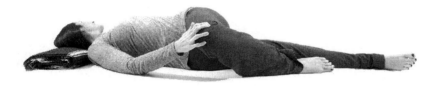

Reclined Knee Down Twist (left knee down, head turned)

INSTRUCTION

- Lie flat on the back with a blanket (long rectangle fold) under the head.
- Keep left leg lengthened and hug the right knee into the chest.
- Step the right foot on the left thigh and use the left hand to draw the right knee to the left, coming into the twist. The foot can stay on the leg or come down to the earth if that's more comfortable.
- Right arm opens out like a wing.
- Both shoulders rest on the earth, but you can roll onto the left hip to maximize the twist.
- Keep the head at center, gazing up, or turn the gaze over the extended arm to take the twist up into the neck.

- Breathe 2-4 minutes on each side.
- To transition to the other side: come back to center with both hips on the earth. Hug left knee in and straighten right leg. Follow same instruction for the left side.
- To release: come back to center, with both hips on the earth, releasing the twist. Feel free to practice Reclined Knee Hug (both knees) to gently stretch and reset the spine to neutral for 5-10 deep breaths.

RECLINED KNEE HUG (BOTH KNEES)

This is a perfect stretch to get length in the low back to relieve compression and built-up tension from sitting, standing or bending too much. It also gently stretches the hips, taking pressure off the low back while improving flexibility and joint mobility in the spine.

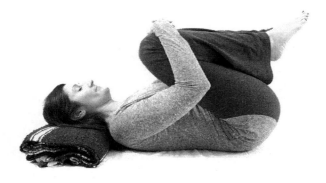

Reclined Knee Hug (hands interlaced over the knees)

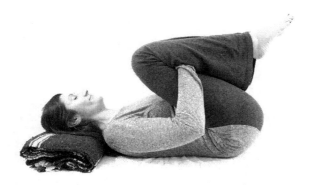

Reclined Knee Hug (hands interlaced under the knees)

INSTRUCTION

- Lie flat on the back with a blanket (long rectangle fold) under the head and knees bent, feet flat on the earth.
- Lift both knees off the earth and hug both knees into the chest, hands interlace over or under the knees.

- Press the low back into the earth as you soften the muscles in the shoulders, neck and face.
- Breathe for 10-20 cycles of breath or longer for a deeper stretch and release.
- To release: let go of the knees and let the feet rest on the earth or lengthen the legs.

RECLINED KNEE HUG (ONE KNEE)

This is a variation and deeper stretch for the hips and low back. As you hug each knee in, soreness in the low back is released; an ideal stretch for releasing tension from too much sitting or standing.

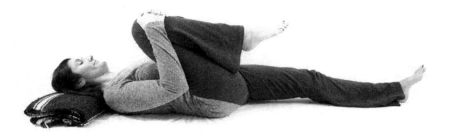

Reclined Knee Hug (hug right knee, hands interlaced over the knee, left leg lengthened)

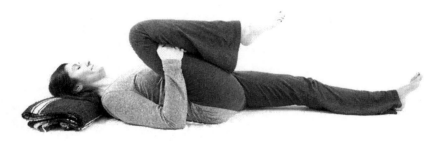

Reclined Knee Hug (hug right knee, hands interlaced under the knee, left leg lengthened)

INSTRUCTION

- Lie flat on the back with a blanket (long rectangle fold) under the head and knees bent, feet flat on the earth.
- Hug the right knee in, interlace the hands over or under the knee. Keep the left leg bent for less stretch or lengthen it out and rest it on the earth for more stretch.
- Soften the shoulders and breathe for 10-20 cycles of breath.
- To transition to the other side: release the right knee and bring the foot flat on the earth. Switch legs and follow instruction for the left side.

- To release: release left knee and keep both knees bent or straighten both legs.

RECLINED PIGEON POSE

This gentle stretch opens the muscles in the back of the hip, buttocks and low back. It targets the same muscles that are gently stretched while practicing Four Part Pigeon and Supported Pigeon Pose. The piriformis muscle softens as stress on the sciatic nerve is reduced.

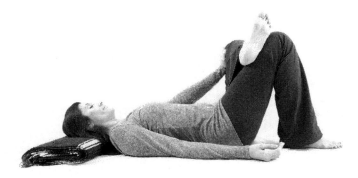

Reclined Pigeon Pose (left foot on right thigh, press left knee away)

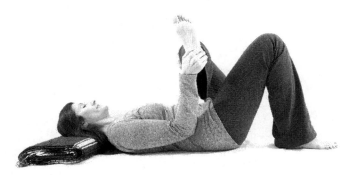

Reclined Pigeon Pose (right hand draws left foot toward the chest as left hand presses left knee away from chest)

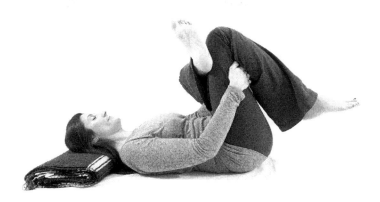

Reclined Pigeon Pose (left foot on right thigh, interlace hands behind thigh and lift foot off the earth for more stretch. Left knee opens away from the chest as left foot is pressed toward the chest)

INSTRUCTION

- Lie flat on the back with a blanket (long rectangle fold) under the head and the knees bent, with the feet flat on the earth.
- Cross the right ankle over the left thigh.
- Strongly press out through the right heel to protect the knee and ankle joints.
- Bring the right hand to the right knee and gently press the knee away, opening the back of the hip.
- For more intensity, grab the right heel with the left hand and lift it off the thigh or interlace the hands behind the thigh and lift the foot off the earth.
- If the opposite foot is lifted, use the thigh as leverage to draw foot in close to the chest as you open the knee away from the chest.
- For all variations, keep the ankle straight and the foot flexed as you draw the foot in toward the chest, while opening the knee away from the chest.
- Breathe 10-20 cycles of breath.

- To transition to the other side: release the leg if it is lifted, uncross the ankle and switch sides, following the same instruction for the left side.
- To release: release the leg if it is lifted, uncross the ankle and bring both feet flat on the earth. Feel free to practice Reclined Knee Hug as you slowly transition.

RECLINED THREE PART HAMSTRING STRETCH

Tight hamstrings pull on the muscles of the low back, creating pain and tension. This series of stretches is a way to stretch open all the parts of the hamstrings to relieve the tension. The back of the leg, including the calf muscles and Achilles tendons, groin, muscles of the outside of the leg and buttocks are stretched as well.

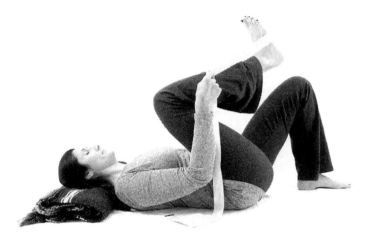

Reclined Three Part Hamstring Stretch Transition (on back with feet flat, knees bent. Blanket, long rectangle fold, under head. Place strap around foot and lengthen leg toward sky)

RECLINED THREE PART HAMSTRING STRETCH: PART ONE

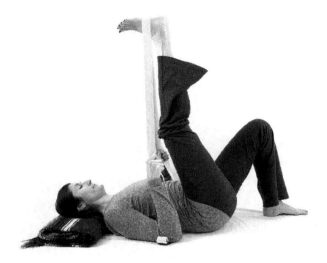

Reclined Three Part Hamstring Stretch (Part One, leg lengthened toward sky)

INSTRUCTION

- Place a strap next to you and lie flat on your back with a blanket (long rectangle fold) under the head with knees bent, feet flat on the earth.
- Hug the right knee into the chest. Place the strap around the foot and lengthen the leg toward the sky.
- Straighten the leg to the best of your ability and press out through the heel.
- Use the strap to guide the toes to the forehead for more intensity. Though the leg may be straight, keep a soft bend in the knee so you are not hyperextending.
- Soften shoulders, jaw and face as you breathe into the back of the leg. Imagine you could send the breath into the stretch to soften and release resistance in the back of the leg.
- Breathe 10-20 cycles of breath.

RECLINED THREE PART HAMSTRING STRETCH: PART TWO

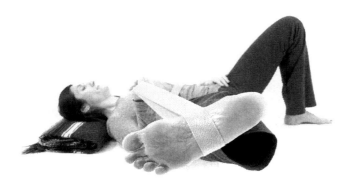

Reclined Three Part Hamstring Stretch (Part Two, open leg out)

INSTRUCTION

- Inhale, grab both straps with the right hand and as you exhale, open the leg out to the right.
- Go to the first place of resistance but not into pain. Keep the leg close to the torso for less intensity. For more intensity, open the leg out further and draw the toes toward the forehead.
- Keep flexing the foot, pressing out through the heel, keeping both hips on the earth.
- Keep a slight bend in the leg to avoid hyperextension.
- Breathe into the stretch in the inside of the leg for 10-20 cycles of breath with a soft jaw and face.

RECLINED THREE PART HAMSTRING STRETCH: PART THREE

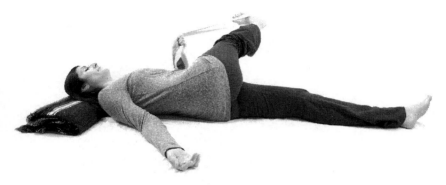

Reclined Three Part Hamstring Stretch (Part Three, cross the right leg to the left)

INSTRUCTION

- Slightly bend the right leg on inhale and use the straps to guide the leg back to center on exhale.
- Inhale, grab both straps with the left hand. Exhale, draw the right leg over to the left on exhale. Feel free to roll onto the left hip.
- Hover the foot over the earth or bring the foot down to the earth. Move the feet closer together for less intensity, and spread the feet further apart for more.
- Both shoulders are resting on the earth.
- Breathe into the stretch on the outside of the leg, hip and low back for 10-20 deep breaths.
- To transition to the other side: slightly bend the leg and use the straps to draw the leg back to center. Bend the knee and remove the strap. Rest right foot flat on the earth and hug the left leg in. Place your strap around the foot and follow instructions for the left side.

- To release: slightly bend the leg and use the straps to draw the leg back to center. Bend the knee and remove the strap. Practice Reclined Knee Hug or lengthen both legs out for a few breaths before you transition.

SEATED FORWARD FOLD

Forward folds are calming to the nervous system and teach surrender. They are also helpful to ease anxiety and this particular forward fold gently stretches the low back, sacrum and back of the hips.

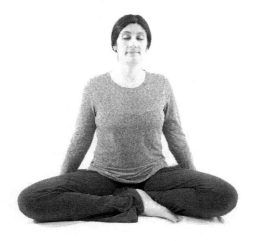

Seated Forward Fold (right leg crossed in front, hands by hips, straight spine, less stretch)

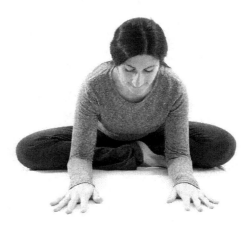

Seated Forward Fold (right leg crossed in front, forearms on earth, straight spine, more stretch)

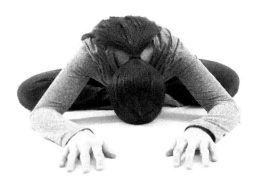

Seated Forward Fold (right leg crossed in front, forehead on earth, round spine, most stretch)

INSTRUCTION

- Come into a comfortable seated position with the right leg crossed in front. Feel free to sit up on a blanket (long rectangle fold) so hips are higher than the knees. This eliminates rounding forward and protects the spine.
- Lengthen the spine, lift the sternum and reach out through the crown of the head while softening the shoulders down.
- Place your hands on the earth, next to the hips, and inhale and as you exhale, hinge the hips forward slightly. Keep your hands by your sides.
- For more stretch and a deeper fold, inhale, find length in the side body and as you exhale, place the hands on the earth in front of you, hinge at the hips and fold.
- Walk the hands out or rest the forearms on the earth. Be sure there is no strain in the neck or shoulders and the fold is coming from the hips. Allow gravity to help you fold deeper, without forcing or tightening the neck and shoulders.
- Keep the spine straight if you have any disk issues or low back tension. Drop the tailbone down to the earth as you reach out

through the crown of the head; the neck is an extension of the spine.
- If there is no injury in the low back or disks, feel free to round the spine, relaxing the neck and shoulders.
- Keep the gaze down as you breathe deeply, lifting the waist out of the hips with each inhale. With each exhale, hinge forward slightly as the hips start to open.
- Breathe slowly and deeply into the hips and legs, softening any tension for 2-4 minutes, as you hold the pose.
- Visualize length and space in the low, mid and upper back as you cascade the breath up and down the spine, releasing any remaining tension between the discs.
- To transition to the other side: come back to a tall spine if you were folding forward. Switch the cross of the legs and follow same instruction for left side.
- To release: bring the torso upright if you were folding forward and uncross the legs. Hands come behind you as legs lengthen out in front of you. Gently rock the legs side to side and circle the ankles.

SEATED PIGEON WITH HALF HERO

This pose combines two very different stretches in the legs to ultimately stretch out tension in the low and mid back sections and in the top of the thighs. Powerful stretches in the back of the hip paired with a strong stretch in the thigh muscle are sure to open up and release stiff and tight muscles.

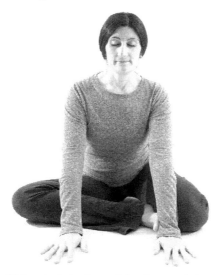

Seated Pigeon with Half Hero (right leg forward, hands on earth forward fold)

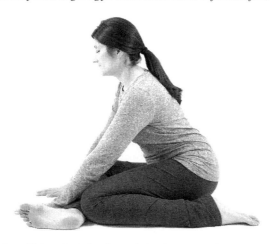

Seated Pigeon with Half Hero (right leg forward, hands on earth forward fold, side view)

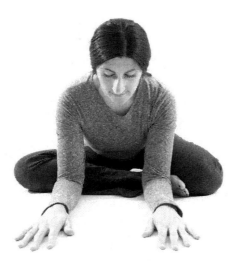

Seated Pigeon with Half Hero (right leg forward, fold onto forearms, straight spine)

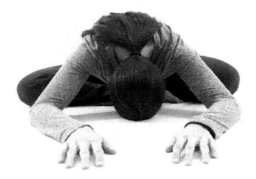

Seated Pigeon with Half Hero (right leg forward, fold onto forearms, round spine)

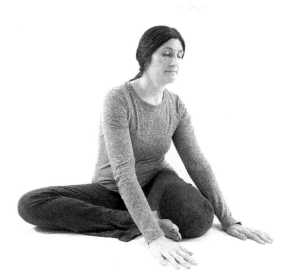

Seated Pigeon with Half Hero (right leg forward, draw hands toward foot)

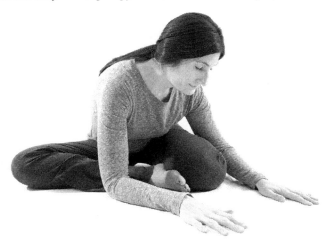

Seated Pigeon with Half Hero (right leg forward, draw forearms toward foot)

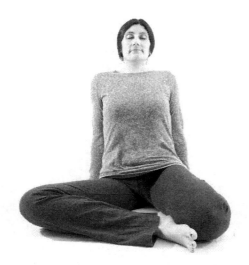

Seated Pigeon with Half Hero (right leg forward, half hero stretch – hands on earth behind hips, chin to chest)

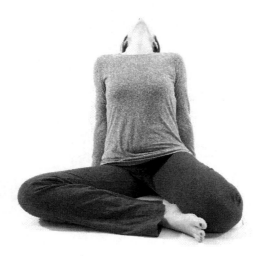

Seated Pigeon with Half Hero (right leg forward, half hero stretch – hands on earth behind hips, head back)

YOGA FOR LOW BACK AND HIP HEALTH

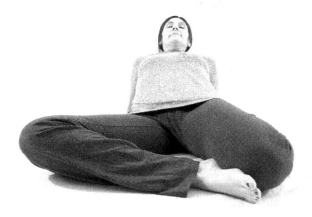

Seated Pigeon with Half Hero (right leg forward, half hero stretch – forearms on earth behind hips, chin to chest)

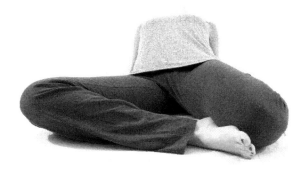

Seated Pigeon with Half Hero (right leg forward, half hero stretch – forearms on earth behind hips, head back)

INSTRUCTION

- From a comfortable cross-legged seated position, take the left foot and tuck it back next to the hip with the knee fully bent.
- Right leg is bent in front, working the shin forward. The further forward the foot, the deeper the stretch.
- Adjust the foot and find the position right for you. Balance the hips as much as possible; even if you need to use a blanket (long rectangle fold or small rectangle fold) under one hip to keep the hips centered.

- Place the hands on the earth in front of you.
- Stay here, or for a deeper stretch, inhale, lengthen the ribs and as you exhale, fold, coming onto the forearms or rest forehead on the earth. Spend about 10-20 cycles of breath here.
- Moving into a deeper stretch for the side of the back, draw the hands or forearms toward the front foot and breathe softly and slowly into the low back and hips for another 10-20 breaths.
- Use an inhale to come up if you are folded forward.
- On exhale, place the hands behind you, moving into the half hero stretch, opening the front of the leg.
- Walk the hands back for more stretch or drop down onto the forearms.
- If you are down on the forearms and the left knee is coming off the earth, come back onto the hands.
- If you're on the forearms and the knee is on the earth, keep the chin tucked so back of neck is long or gaze back, releasing the neck to open the throat center (**do not attempt if there is currently or any history of a neck injury**).
- Gently draw the navel down to the spine.
- Breathe into the front of the leg for 10-20 breaths.
- Use an inhale to tuck the chin back toward the chest if the neck was back. Engage the core and come back up if you were down on the elbows.
- To transition to the other side: bring the left leg forward and tuck the right heel back by the buttocks. Follow the instruction for the left side.
- To release: bring back leg forward and stretch both legs out in front out you. Hands come behind and gently rock the legs side to side and circle the ankles.

SEATED SIDE BEND

Lateral movements are helpful to relieve tension in the hips, low back and muscles along the side body including the ribs and shoulders. Side bends open breathing muscles, making deep breaths more accessible.

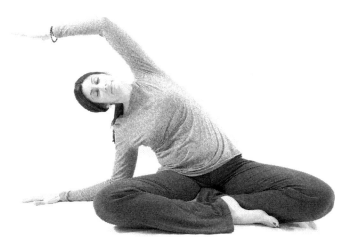

Seated Side Bend (bending toward the right, opening the left side, head neutral)

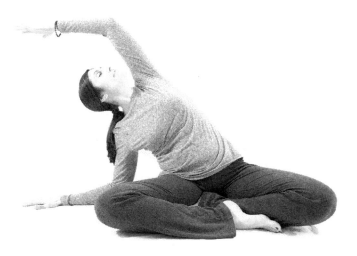

Seated Side Bend (bending toward the right, opening the left side, gaze up)

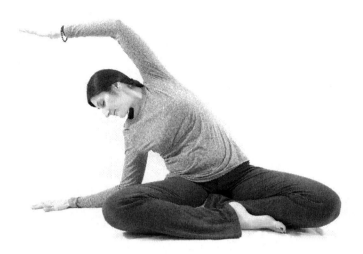

Seated Side Bend (bending toward the right, opening the left side, gaze down)

INSTRUCTION

- Come into a comfortable seated position with the legs crossed. Feel free to sit up on a blanket (long rectangle fold) so hips are higher than the knees. This eliminates rounding forward and protects the spine.
- Place the right hand down on the earth about 12 inches away from the hip. Fingers point away from the hip.
- Inhale the left arm up and exhale the arm overhead as you slide the bottom hand out.
- Drop the right shoulder down away from the ear and bend the right elbow.
- Gaze down at the earth for less stretch in the neck, keep the head neutral, with the ear stacked over the shoulder, or gaze up at top arm for more stretch in the neck.
- Use your inhales to roll the chest open and your exhales to reach out through the fingers, rolling the right side of the heart up toward sky.

- If the arm overhead is too intense, bring the left hand behind the back and roll the left shoulder back to open the chest.
- Breathe slow and deep for 10-20 cycles of breath, softening with each exhale.
- To transition to other side: inhale both arms up through center, exhale hands to heart center. Switch the cross of the legs. Follow these instructions for the left side.
- To release: inhale and draw the torso back to center releasing the side bend.

SEATED TWIST

An easy seated twist to unwind tension in the hips, spine and neck, while gently detoxing organs.

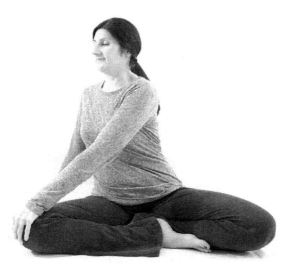

Seated Twist (twisting toward the right, chin parallel with the chest)

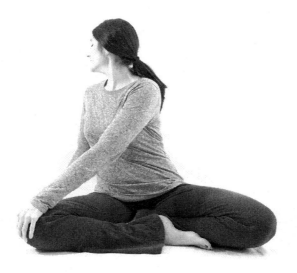

Seated Twist (twisting toward the right, gaze over back shoulder)

INSTRUCTION

- Come into a comfortable seated position with the legs crossed. Feel free to sit up on a blanket (long rectangle fold) so hips are higher than the knees. This eliminates rounding forward and protects the spine.
- Inhale, lengthen the arms up toward sky, finding length in the side body and as you exhale, twist to the right, bringing the left hand on the right knee and right hand or fingertips to the earth. Shoulders parallel.
- Be sure the twist is coming from the torso, not the shoulders.
- Use inhales to lengthen and exhales to deepen the twist.
- Keep the chin parallel with the chest or gaze over the back shoulder to take the twist into the neck. **If there is an history of injury or any injury in the neck, keep the chin parallel to the chest.**
- Breathe slowly and deeply for 10-20 cycles of breath, softening with each exhale.
- To transition to the other side: inhale back to center and switch the cross of the legs. Follow instruction for the left side.
- To release: inhale and draw the torso back to center, releasing the twist.

SIDE LYING QUAD STRETCH

Stretching open the large muscles of the thigh in this extremely gentle way helps to realign the pelvis and release tension in the front of the hip and leg. This stretch is also beneficial for the knee and ankle joints.

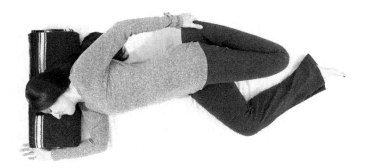

Side Lying Quad Stretch

INSTRUCTION

- Lie flat on the back with a blanket (long rectangle fold) under the head and knees bent, feet flat on the earth.
- Slowly lie on your right side.
- Bend the left leg, reach back and grab the top of the foot. If the foot isn't accessible, place a strap around the foot and draw the strap close to the buttocks.
- Keep the right leg straight or bend it.
- Draw the left foot in close to the buttocks, stretching open the front of the thigh. For more stretch, draw the knee slightly back but be sure you are not feeling any pain in the knee.
- Soften the shoulders and breathe into the stretch in the front of the thigh.
- Hold for 1-2 minutes.

- To transition to the other side: gently release the left foot and roll flat on the back. Without rushing and being mindfully aware of movements, slowly roll onto the left side. Follow instructions for the right side.
- To release: gently release the foot and take a few breaths on your side before transitioning.

TABLE POSE

This pose is a neutral position for the spine to rest in and reset.

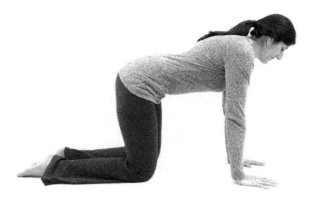

Table Pose (neutral spine)

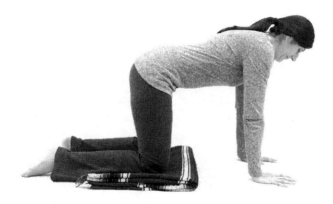

Table Pose (neutral spine, blanket, large rectangle fold, under knees)

INSTRUCTION

- Come onto hands and knees. If there is discomfort in the knees, place a blanket (large rectangle fold or long rectangle fold) under knees for padding.
- Stack wrists under shoulders and keep knees under hips.
- Keep the gaze down and reach out through the crown of the head as you lift out through the shoulders.
- Visualize a long spine from the tailbone to the crown.

- If the wrists are bothering you, make fists with the hands or use a small blanket roll under the palms and fingers.

FOUR PART PIGEON

This series of poses is a slower release of tension in the hip and back. It is helpful to relieve piriformis syndrome, sciatic nerve pain and stretch tense muscles from sitting or standing too much.

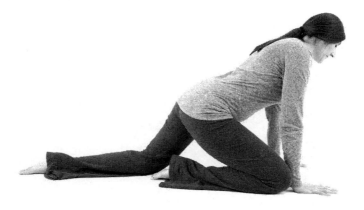

Four Part Pigeon Transition (draw right knee to right wrist as left leg strats to lengthen back)

FOUR PART PIGEON: PART ONE

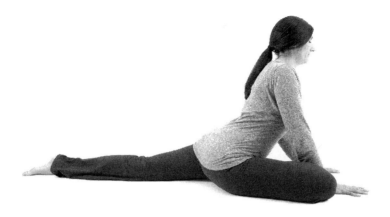

Four Part Pigeon (Part One, hands on earth)

INSTRUCTION

- Come into Table Pose. (Have a bolster, blankets and a block nearby if you would like to transition to Supported Pigeon for Part Four.)
- Draw the right knee to the right wrist. Draw the right foot to the left as you lengthen the left leg back. Move the heel closer to the groin for less intensity or away from the groin for more.
- Spread the fingers wide and stack the wrists under the shoulders.
- Stay on hands and continue to center the hips.
- Breathe for 2-4 minutes. Soften the face, jaw, shoulders and hands as you gaze down or close the eyes.
- Imagine you can breathe down into the hips and exhale out tension.

FOUR PART PIGEON: PART TWO

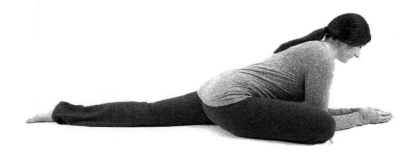

Four Part Pigeon (Part Two, forearms on earth)

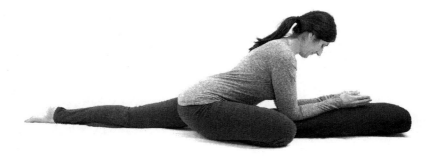

Four Part Pigeon (Part Two, forearms on bolster)

INSTRUCTION

- Using an exhale, fold down onto the forearms. Use a bolster or a block under the forearms if forearms on the earth is too much stretch.
- Interlace the hands, press the palms together or keep the palms flat on the earth or bolster. Soften any clenching in the hands, face or jaw as you breathe deeply.
- Draw the ribs forward, lifting them out of the waist as you breathe slowly for 2-4 minutes.

FOUR PART PIGEON: PART THREE

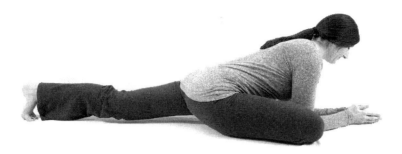

Four Part Pigeon (Part Three, tuck toes under and lift back knee off the earth)

INSTRUCTION

- Staying on forearms, tuck the left toes under and lift the left knee slightly off the earth. Lift the thighbone up as you lengthen the leg back.
- This stretches the front of the left hip flexor.
- Breathe for 6-8 cycles of breath, then gently place the knee down and untuck the toes, resting the top of the foot on the earth.

FOUR PART PIGEON: PART FOUR

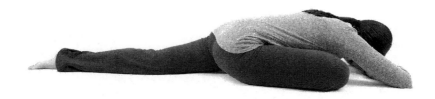

Four Part Pigeon (Part Four, forward fold, forehead on forearms)

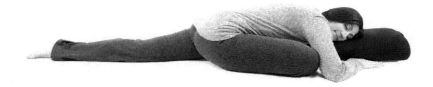

Four Part Pigeon (Part Four, forward fold into Supported Pigeon Pose)

INSTRUCTION

- Once the back knee is down, you can fold deeper, bringing the forehead down onto the forearms, the earth or set up your props and transition to Supported Pigeon Pose.
- Hold for 10-20 slow cycles of breath or longer for more stretch.
- To transition to the other side: come into Table Pose. Practice Modified Downward Facing Dog or Downward Facing Dog, "walk the dog," to stretch out the compression in the right leg. Come back to Table Pose and follow instructions for all four parts on the left side.
- To release: come back onto hands and slowly make your way back into Table Pose. Practice Modified Downward Facing Dog or Downward Facing Dog, "walking the dog," to stretch out the compression in the left leg.

CHAPTER FOUR

YOGA SEQUENCES

SEQUENCE #1

Ease Low Back Pain

Gentle Yoga (short sequence)

1. Begin with **Reclined Knee Hug (both knees)** for 5-10 slow breaths.
2. When you are ready, transition to **Reclined Knee Hug (one knee)** and breathe, hugging each knee in for 10 cycles of breath, mindfully alternating the knees while gently stretching the hips and low back.
3. Release the knees and come into **Reclined ½ Crescent**, holding each side for 3-5 minutes.
4. Bring the body back to center and take a full-body stretch from the fingers to the toes. Slowly come onto one side and practice **Side Lying Quad Stretch**. Hold each side for 1-2 minutes.
5. When you are ready, gently come onto the back once more and transition to **Reclined Knee Down Twist**. Practice this twist and hold 3-5 minutes, each side, gently unwinding the spine.
6. Slowly hug the knees into the chest for **Reclined Knee Hug (both knees)**.
7. Place a bolster under the knees and lengthen the legs out, resting the heels on the earth for **Supported Final Relaxation**.

SEQUENCE #1 (continued)

Ease Low Back Pain

Gentle Yoga (short sequence)

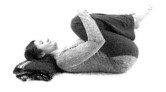

1. Reclined Knee Hug (both knees)   2. Reclined Knee Hug (one knee)

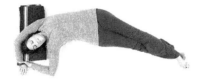

3. Reclined ½ Crescent   4. Side Lying Quad Stretch

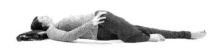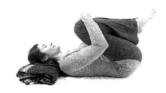

5. Reclined Knee Down Twist   6. Reclined Knee Hug (both knees)

SEQUENCE #1 (continued)
Ease Low Back Pain
Gentle Yoga (short sequence)

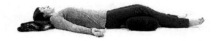

7. Supported Final Relaxation

SEQUENCE #2

Ease Low Back Pain

Gentle Yoga (long sequence)

1. Practice **Seated Side Bend** for 10-20 cycles of breaths.
2. Return the spine to neutral and come into a **Seated Twist**. Hold pose for 10-20 breaths.
3. Come back to a neutral spine, lengthen the side body and come into a **Seated Forward Fold**, holding for 2-4 minutes. Release the fold and **switch the cross of the legs. REPEAT Seated Side Bend, Seated Twist and Seated Forward Fold on the other side.**
4. Transition into **Seated Pigeon with Half Hero**. Practice on both sides for 10-20 breaths each in the forward fold and reclined half hero stretch.
5. Slowly make your way onto hands and knees for **Table Pose**. Practice 5-10 rounds of **Cat/Cow Tilts** to gently loosen tension in the spine.
6. After your last round, come back to **Table Pose** and bring the right foot between the hands for **Low Lunge Hands On Thigh**. Keep shifting the hips forward and breathe deeply for 20-30 cycles of breath on each side.
7. Come back into **Table Pose** and practice **Child's Pose** for 10-20 cycles of breath.
8. Gracefully release the foot and practice **Modified Downward Facing Dog** or **Downward Facing Dog**, "walking the dog," until the right leg feels stretched out.

SEQUENCE #2 (continued)

Ease Low Back Pain

Gentle Yoga (long sequence)

9. Transition into **Reclined Knee Hug (both knees)**. Hold the pose for 10-20 cycles of breath.
10. Hug the right knee in and practice **Reclined Knee Hug (one knee)**. Hold the pose for 10-20 cycles of breath.
11. Grab your strap and place it around the right foot, moving into **Reclined Three Part Hamstring Stretch**. Practice 10-20 cycles of breath each part.
12. Practice **Hip Circles** after the third part of the hamstring stretch for 10-20 cycles of breath. **REPEAT Reclined Knee Hug (one knee), Reclined Three Part Hamstring Stretch and Hip Circles** on the left side.
13. Remove the strap and come into **Reclined Pigeon Pose**. Hold 10-20 breaths each side.
14. Transition into **Reclined Knee Down Twist** for 2-4 minutes each side.
15. Slowly hug the knees into the chest for **Reclined Knee Hug (both knees)**.
16. Place a bolster under the knees and lengthen the legs out, resting the heels on the earth for **Supported Final Relaxation**.

SEQUENCE #2 (continued)

Ease Low Back Pain
Gentle Yoga (long sequence)

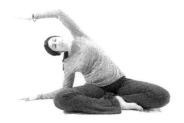

1. Seated Side Bend

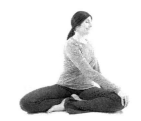

2. Seated Twist

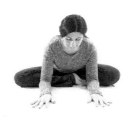

3. Seated Forward Fold

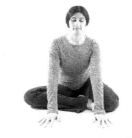

4. Seated Pigeon with Half Hero

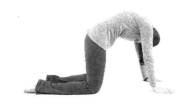

5. Cat/Cow Tilts

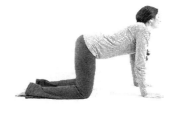

5. Cat/Cow Tilts

SEQUENCE #2 (continued)
Ease Low Back Pain
Gentle Yoga (long sequence)

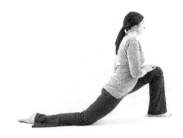

6. Low Lunge Hands on Thigh

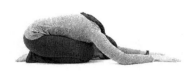

7. Child's Pose

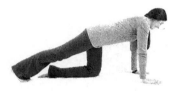

8. Modified Downward Facing Dog

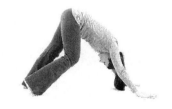

8. Downward Facing Dog (walking the dog)

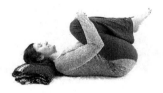

9. Reclined Knee Hug (Both Knees)

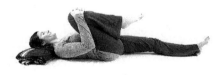

10. Reclined Knee Hug (one knee)

SEQUENCE #2 (continued)
Ease Low Back Pain
Gentle Yoga (long sequence)

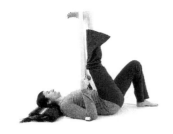

11. Reclined Three Part Hamstring Stretch (Part One)

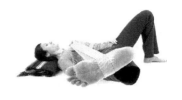

11. Reclined Three Part Hamstring Stretch (Part Two)

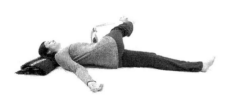

11. Reclined Three Part Hamstring Stretch (Part Three)

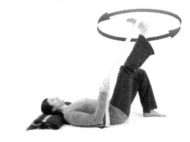

12. Hip Circles

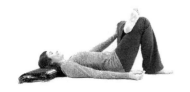

13. Reclined Pigeon Pose

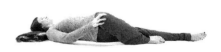

14. Reclined Knee Down Twist

SEQUENCE #2 (continued)

Ease Low Back Pain

Gentle Yoga (long sequence)

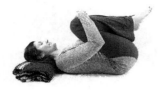

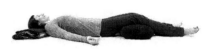

15. Reclined Knee Hug (both knees)

16. Supported Final Relaxation

SEQUENCE #3

Ease Low Back Pain

Restorative Yoga (short sequence)

1. Practice **Supported Reclining Pose** for 5-10 minutes depending on desired stretch. Before you release, lengthen the arms back and hold onto opposite elbows or forearms for 5-10 breaths. Slowly float the arms down and rest them by your side. Bend legs and mindfully rock knees side to side. Transition to the forearm on one side and slowly press up to seated.
2. Come into **Table Pose** and practice 5-8 rounds of **Cat/Cow Tilts**.
3. From a neutral spine, move into **Supported Child's Pose**. Practice 3 minutes, turn the head, practice 3 more minutes.
4. Release **Supported Child's Pose** and practice **Modified Downward Facing Dog** or **Downward Facing Dog**, "walking the dog," until the right leg feels stretched out.
5. Slowly come onto the back and practice **Reclined ½ Crescent**. Hold for 3-5 minutes each side.
6. Bring knees back to center and practice **Reclined Knee Hug (both knees)** for 5-10 deep breaths.
7. When you are ready, practice **Supported Final Relaxation** for 5-10 minutes.

SEQUENCE #3 (continued)
Ease Low Back Pain
Restorative Yoga (short sequence)

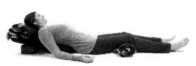

1. *Supported Reclining Pose*

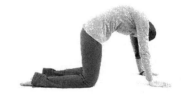

2. *Cat/Cow Tilts*

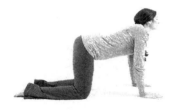

2. *Cat/Cow Tilts*

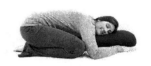

3. *Supported Child's Pose*

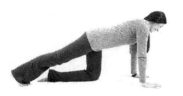

4. *Modified Downward Facing Dog*

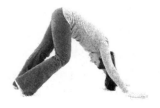

4. *Downward Facing Dog (walking the dog)*

SEQUENCE #3 (continued)

Ease Low Back Pain

Restorative Yoga (short sequence)

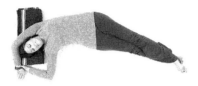

5. Reclined ½ Crescent

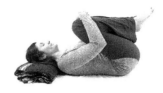

6. Reclined Knee Hug (both knees)

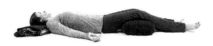

7. Supported Final Relaxation

SEQUENCE #4

Ease Low Back Pain
Restorative Yoga (long sequence)

1. Practice **Supported Reclining Pose** for 5-10 minutes depending on desired stretch. Before you release, lengthen the arms back and hold onto opposite elbows or forearms for 5-10 breaths. Slowly float the arms down and rest them by your side. Bend legs and mindfully rock knees side to side. Transition to the forearm on one side and slowly press up to seated.
2. Come into **Table Pose** and practice 5-8 rounds of **Cat/Cow Tilts**.
3. From a neutral spine, move into **Supported Child's Pose**. Practice 3 minutes, turn the head, practice 3 more minutes.
4. Release **Supported Child's Pose** and practice **Modified Downward Facing Dog** or **Downward Facing Dog**, "walking the dog," until the right leg feels stretched out.
5. Set up for **Supported ½ Moon** and breathe deeply for 6-8 minutes each side. Before releasing, practice **Arm Circles** for 10-20 cycles of breath.
6. Adjust the bolster and practice **Supported Belly Down Twist** for 6-8 minutes each side.
7. Transition to **Reclined Knee Hug (both knees)**. Breathe in stillness, pressing the low back into the earth for 5-10 cycles of breath.
8. Release the knees and practice **Supported Final Relaxation** for 5-10 minutes.

SEQUENCE #4 (continued)

Ease Low Back Pain
Restorative Yoga (long sequence)

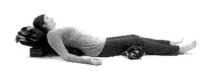

1. Supported Reclining Pose

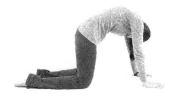

2. Cat/Cow Tilts

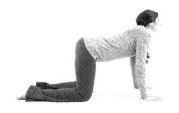

2. Cat/Cow Tilts

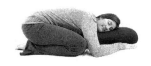

3. Supported Child's Pose

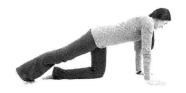

4. Modified Downward Facing Dog

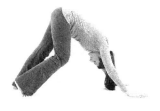

4. Downward Facing Dog (walking the dog)

SEQUENCE #4 (continued)
Ease Low Back Pain
Restorative Yoga (long sequence)

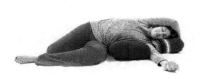

5. Supported ½ Moon

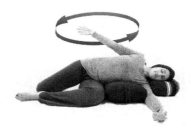

5. Arm Circles

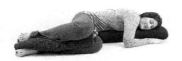

6. Supported Belly Down Twist

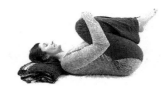

7. Reclined Knee Hug (both knees)

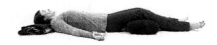

8. Supported Final Relaxation

SEQUENCE #5

Ease Hip Tension

Gentle Yoga (short sequence)

1. Come into **Table Pose** and practice 5-8 rounds of **Cat/Cow Tilts**.
2. From a neutral spine, step the right foot between the hands for **Low Lunge Hands on Thigh.** Hold for 20-30 breaths.
3. Bring hands back to the earth and move into **Four Part Pigeon**. Hold parts one and two for 2-4 minutes depending on level of intensity and part three for 6-8 slow breaths. Practice part four for 10-20 deep breaths. Stay connected to the stretch in the hip.
4. Practice **Modified Downward Facing Dog** or **Downward Facing Dog**, "walking the dog," until the right leg feels stretched out. REPEAT **Low Lunge Hands on Thigh, Four Part Pigeon** and **Modified Downward Facing Dog** or **Downward Facing Dog**, "walking the dog," on the left side.
5. Come into a comfortable seated position and move into **Seated Forward Fold.** Hold each side 15-20 breaths.
6. Slowly transition to **Reclined Knee Hug (both knees)** for 10 cycles of breath.
7. Keep right knee hugged in as you release left knee and practice **Reclined Knee Hug (one knee)** for 10-20 slow breaths.
8. Place your strap around the right foot and move into **Hip Circles** for 10-20 breaths.
9. Transition into **Reclined Knee Down Twist** for 2-4 minutes. REPEAT **Reclined Knee Hug (one knee), Hip Circles** and **Reclined Knee Down Twist** on the left side.
10. Practice **Supported Final Relaxation** for 5-10 minutes.

SEQUENCE #5 (continued)
Ease Hip Tension
Gentle Yoga (short sequence)

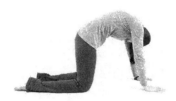

1. Cat/Cow Tilts

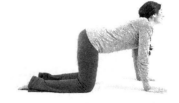

1. Cat/Cow Tilts

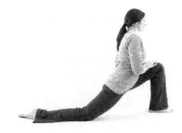

2. Low Lunge Hands on Thigh

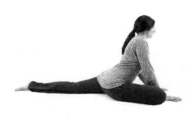

3. Four Part Pigeon (Part One)

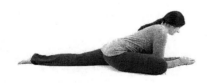

3. Four Part Pigeon (Part Two)

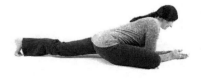

3. Four Part Pigeon (Part Three)

SEQUENCE #5 (continued)
Ease Hip Tension
Gentle Yoga (short sequence)

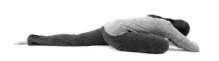
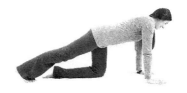

3. Four Part Pigeon (Part Four)

4. Modified Downward Facing Dog

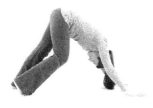
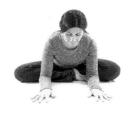

4. Downward Facing Dog (walking the dog)

5. Seated Forward Fold

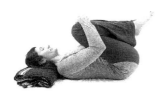
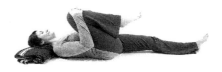

6. Reclined Knee Hug (both knees)

7. Reclined Knee Hug (one knee)

SEQUENCE #5 (continued)
Ease Hip Tension
Gentle Yoga (short sequence)

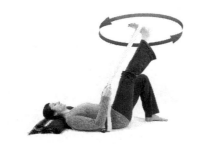
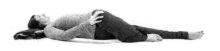

8. Hip Circles   *9. Reclined Knee Down Twist*

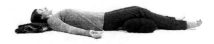

10. Supported Final Relaxation

SEQUENCE #6

Ease Hip Tension

Gentle Yoga (long sequence)

1. Practice **Reclined Leg Rest** and breathe deeply for 5-10 minutes.
2. Transition to **Reclined Knee Hug (both knees)** for 10-20 cycles of breath.
3. Keep right knee hugged in and practice **Reclined Knee Hug (one knee)** for 5-10 cycles of breath.
4. Place your strap around the right foot and transition to **Reclined Three Part Hamstring Stretch**. Hold each part for 10-20 cycles of breath.
5. Move into **Hip Circles** for 10-20 cycles of breath. **REPEAT Reclined Knee Hug (one knee), Reclined Three Part Hamstring Stretch** and **Hip Circles** on the left side.
6. Slowly come into **Table Pose** and move into **Cat/Cow Tilts**. Take 5-10 rounds.
7. From a neutral spine, step the right foot between the hands for **Low Lunge Hands on Thigh**. Hold for 20-30 breaths, drawing the hips forward.
8. Bring hands back to the earth and move into **Four Part Pigeon**. Hold parts one and two for 2-4 minutes depending on level of intensity and part three for 6-8 slow breaths. Practice part four 10-20 deep breaths. Stay connected to the stretch in the hip.
9. **Practice Modified Downward Facing Dog** or **Downward Facing Dog**, "walking the dog," until the right leg feels stretched out. REPEAT **Low Lunge Hands on Thigh, Four Part Pigeon** and **Modified Downward Facing Dog** or **Downward Facing Dog** on the left side.

SEQUENCE #6 (continued)
Ease Hip Tension
Gentle Yoga (long sequence)

10. Transition into **Seated Pigeon with Half Hero**. Practice on both sides for 10-20 breaths each in the forward fold and reclined half hero stretch.
11. Slowly come onto the back and practice **Reclined Knee Hug (both knees)** for 10 cycles of breath.
12. Have your bolster nearby and move into **Supported Bridge With Bent Legs**. Hold 3-5 minutes.
13. Ground the feet down and slowly lift the hips up and remove the bolster. Lengthen the low back and lower the hips down. **Practice Reclined Knee Hug (both knees)** for 10 slow cycles of breath.
14. Release the knees and transition to **Reclined Knee Down Twist** for 3-5 minutes each side.
15. Practice **Supported Final Relaxation** for 5-10 minutes.

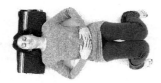

1. Reclined Leg Rest

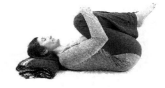

2. Reclined Knee Hug (both knees)

SEQUENCE #6 (continued)

Ease Hip Tension
Gentle Yoga (long sequence)

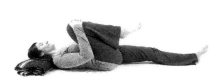

3. Reclined Knee Hug (one knee)

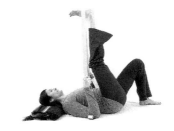

4. Reclined Three Part Hamstring Stretch (Part One)

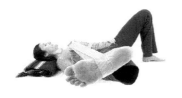

4. Reclined Three Part Hamstring Stretch (Part Two)

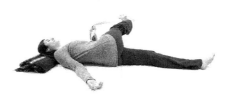

4. Reclined Three Part Hamstring Stretch (Part Three)

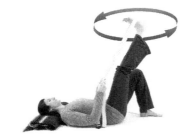

5. Hip Circles

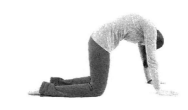

6. Cat/Cow Tilts

SEQUENCE #6 (continued)
Ease Hip Tension
Gentle Yoga (long sequence)

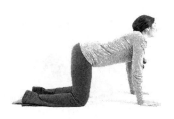

6. Cat/Cow Tilts

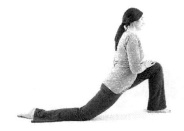

7. Low Lunge Hands on Thigh

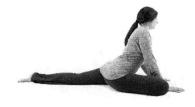

8. Four Part Pigeon (Part One)

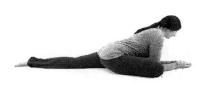

8. Four Part Pigeon (Part Two)

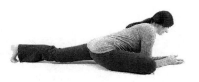

8. Four Part Pigeon (Part Three)

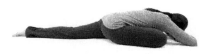

8. Four Part Pigeon (Part Four)

SEQUENCE #6 (continued)

Ease Hip Tension
Gentle Yoga (long sequence)

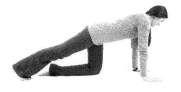

9. Modified Downward Facing Dog

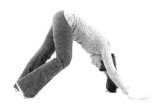

9. Downward Facing Dog (walking the dog)

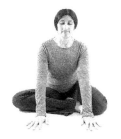

10. Seated Pigeon with Half Hero

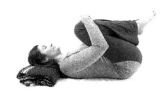

11. Reclined Knee Hug (both knees)

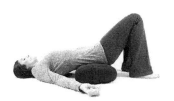

12. Supported Bridge with Bent Legs

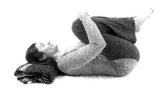

13. Reclined Knee Hug (both knees)

SEQUENCE #6 (continued)
Ease Hip Tension
Gentle Yoga (long sequence)

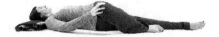 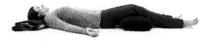

14. Reclined Knee Down Twist   *15. Supported Final Relaxation*

SEQUENCE #7

Ease Hip Tension

Restorative Yoga (short sequence)

1. Practice **Reclined Leg Rest** and breathe deeply for 5-10 minutes.
2. Transition into **Supported Bridge With Bent Legs**. Hold 3-5 minutes.
3. Release and move into **Reclined Knee Hug (both knees)** for 10 slow cycles of breath.
4. Come into **Table Pose** and practice 5-8 rounds of **Cat/Cow Tilts**.
5. From a neutral spine, move into **Supported Child's Pose**. Practice 3 minutes, turn the head, practice 3 more minutes.
6. Release **Supported Child's Pose** and practice **Modified Downward Facing Dog** or **Downward Facing Dog**, "walking the dog." Stretch until the back of the legs feel open.
7. When you are ready, set up your props and move into **Supported Belly Down Twist with Extended Legs Variation**. Practice each side for 5-8 minutes.
8. Practice **Supported Inversion** for 8-10 minutes.

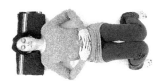

1. Reclined Leg Rest

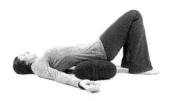

2. Supported Bridge with Bent Legs

SEQUENCE #7 (continued)

Ease Hip Tension

Restorative Yoga (short sequence)

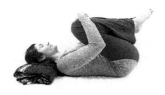

3. Reclined Knee Hug (both knees)

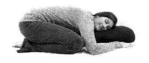

4. Cat/Cow Tilts

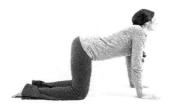

4. Cat/Cow Tilts

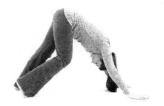

5. Supported Child's Pose

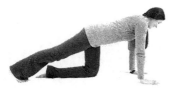

6. Modified Downward Facing Dog

6. Downward Facing Dog (walking the dog)

SEQUENCE #7 (continued)

Ease Hip Tension

Restorative Yoga (short sequence)

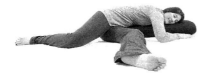
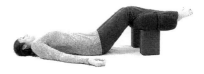

7. *Supported Belly Down Twist (Extended Legs Variation)*

8. *Supported Inversion*

SEQUENCE #8

Ease Hip Tension

Restorative Yoga (long sequence)

1. Practice **Supported Final Relaxation** for 5-10 minutes.
2. Come onto hands and knees and practice 5-8 rounds of **Cat/Cow Tilts**.
3. From a neutral spine, move into **Supported Child's Pose**. Practice 3-4 minutes, turn the head, practice 3-4 more minutes.
4. Release **Supported Child's Pose** and practice **Modified Downward Facing Dog** or **Downward Facing Dog, "walking the dog."** Stretch until the back of the legs feel open.
5. Transition to **Supported ½ Moon**. Practice 6-8 minutes on each side.
6. Come into **Table Pose** and set up for **Supported Pigeon Pose**. Hold 3-6 minutes each side practicing **Modified Downward Facing Dog** or **Downward Facing Dog, "walking the dog"** after each side to release the legs.
7. Come onto the back with your strap nearby and practice **Reclined Three Part Hamstring Stretch** on the right side, holding each part for 10-20 cycles of breath.
8. After part three of the stretch, move into **Hip Circles** for 10-20 cycles of breath. **REPEAT Reclined Three Part Hamstring Stretch** and **Hip Circles** on the left side.
9. Practice **Supported Inversion** for 8-10 minutes.

SEQUENCE #8 (continued)

Ease Hip Tension
Restorative yoga (long sequence)

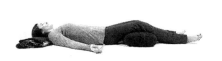

1. Supported Final Relaxation

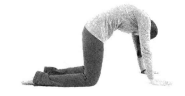

2. Cat/Cow Tilts

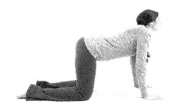

2. Cat/Cow Tilts

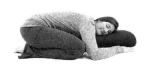

3. Supported Child's Pose

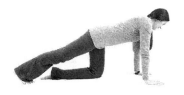

4. Modified Downward Facing Dog

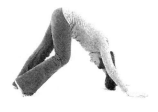

4. Downward Facing Dog (walking the dog)

SEQUENCE #8 (continued)

Ease Hip Tension

Restorative yoga (long sequence)

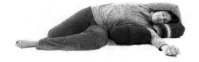 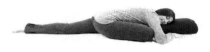

5. Supported ½ Moon   6. Supported Pigeon Pose

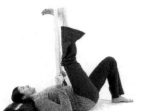 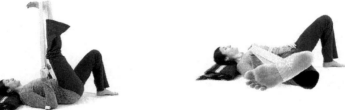

7. Reclined Three Part Hamstring Stretch (Part One)   7. Reclined Three Part Hamstring Stretch (Part Two)

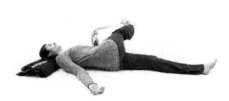 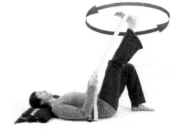

7. Reclined Three Part Hamstring Stretch (Part Three)   8. Hip Circles

SEQUENCE #8 (continued)

Ease Hip Tension

Restorative yoga (long sequence)

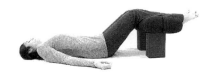

9. Supported Inversion

SEQUENCE #9

Sequence for Piriformis Syndrome/Sciatic Nerve Pain
Gentle and Restorative Yoga (short sequence)

1. Come into **Table Pose** and slowly come onto the belly for **Belly Down ½ Frog** for 2-4 minutes each side.
2. Slowly come back into **Table Pose** and practice **Cat/Cow Tilts** for 10-15 rounds.
3. Come to a neutral spine and step the right foot between the hands for **Low Lunge Hands on Thigh**. Take 20-30 cycles of slow breaths, drawing the hips forward.
4. Move into **Four Part Pigeon** on the right side. Hold parts one and two for 2-4 minutes depending on level of intensity and part three for 6-8 slow breaths. Practice part four for 10-20 slow breaths. Stay connected to the stretch in the hip. **REPEAT Low Lunge Hands on Thigh** and **Four Part Pigeon** on the left side.
5. Transition to **Reclined ½ Crescent**, breathing slowly for 3-5 minutes each side.
6. Come onto one side and move into **Side Lying Quad Stretch** and practice for 10-20 cycles of breath, drawing the foot into the buttocks.
7. Slowly transition and practice **Reclined Knee Down Twist** for 2-4 minutes.
8. Transition to **Reclined Knee Hug (both knees)** for 10-20 cycles of breath.
9. Practice **Supported Inversion** for 8-10 minutes.

SEQUENCE #9 (continued)

Sequence for Piriformis Syndrome/Sciatic Nerve Pain
Gentle and Restorative Yoga (short sequence)

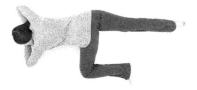

1. Belly Down ½ Frog

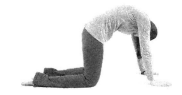

2. Cat/Cow Tilts

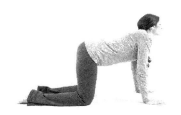

2. Cat/Cow Tilts

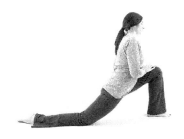

3. Low Lunge Hands on Thigh

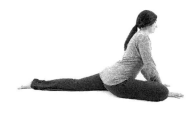

4. Four Part Pigeon (Part One)

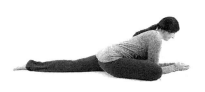

4. Four Part Pigeon (Part Two)

SEQUENCE #9 (continued)
Sequence for Piriformis Syndrome/Sciatic Nerve Pain
Gentle and Restorative Yoga (short sequence)

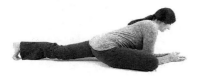

4. Four Part Pigeon (Part Three)

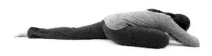

4. Four Part Pigeon (Part Four)

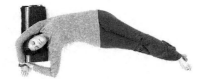

5. Reclined ½ Crescent

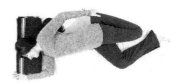

6. Side Lying Quad Stretch

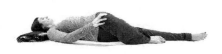

7. Reclined Knee Down Twist

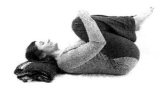

8. Reclined Knee Hug (both knees)

SEQUENCE #9 (continued)
Sequence for Piriformis Syndrome/Sciatic Nerve Pain
Gentle and Restorative Yoga (short sequence)

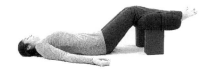

9. Supported Inversion

SEQUENCE #10

Sequence for Piriformis Syndrome/Sciatic Nerve Pain
Gentle and Restorative Yoga (long sequence)

1. Practice **Supported Inversion** for 8-10 minutes.
2. Transition to **Reclined Knee Hug (both knees)** for 10-20 cycles of breath.
3. Come into **Table Pose** and slowly come onto the belly for **Belly Down ½ Frog** for 2-4 minutes each side.
4. Slowly transition back into **Table Pose** and set up for **Supported Belly Down Twist With Extended Legs Variation**. Practice each side for 5-8 minutes.
5. Move into **Four Part Pigeon** on the right side. Hold parts one and two for 2-4 minutes depending on level of intensity and part three for 6-8 slow breaths. Practice part four for 10-20 cycles of breath. Stay connected to the stretch in the hip. Practice **Modified Downward Facing Dog** or **Downward Facing Dog**, "walking the dog," after each side to release the legs.
6. Transition into **Supported Bridge With Bent Legs**. Slowly breathe for 3-5 minutes.
7. Gently remove the bolster and practice **Reclined Knee Hug (both knees)** for 10-20 cycles of breath.
8. Transition to **Reclined ½ Crescent**, practicing each side for 3-5 minutes.
9. Mindfully transition and practice **Side Lying Quad Stretch** for 10-20 cycles of breath, each side.
10. Come into **Reclined Knee Down Twist** for 2-4 minutes, hugging the right knee in.
11. Practice **Reclined Pigeon Pose** on the right side for 10-20 cycles of breath.

SEQUENCE #10 (continued)
Sequence for Piriformis Syndrome/Sciatic Nerve Pain
Gentle and Restorative Yoga (long sequence)

12. Place your strap around the right foot and practice **Hip Circles** for 10-20 cycles of breath. **REPEAT Reclined Knee Down Twist, Reclined Pigeon Pose** and **Hip Circles** on the left side.
13. Practice **Reclined Leg Rest** for 5-10 minutes.

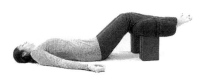

1. Supported Inversion

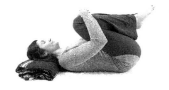

2. Reclined Knee Hug (both knees)

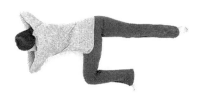

3. Belly Down ½ Frog

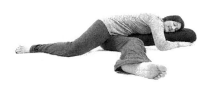

4. Supported Belly Down Twist (Extended Legs Variation)

SEQUENCE #10 (continued)
Sequence for Piriformis Syndrome/Sciatic Nerve Pain
Gentle and Restorative Yoga (long sequence)

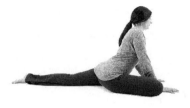

5. Four Part Pigeon (Part One)

5. Four Part Pigeon (Part Two)

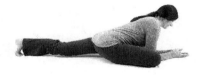

5. Four Part Pigeon (Part Three)

5. Four Part Pigeon (Part Four)

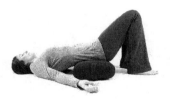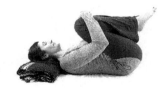

6. Supported Bridge with Bent Legs

7. Reclined Knee Hug (both knees)

SEQUENCE #10 (continued)

Sequence for Piriformis Syndrome/Sciatic Nerve Pain
Gentle and Restorative Yoga (long sequence)

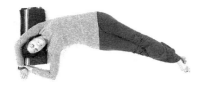

8. Reclined ½ Crescent

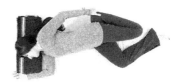

9. Side Lying Quad Stretch

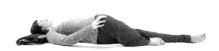

10. Reclined Knee Down Twist

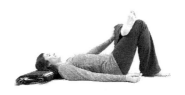

11. Reclined Pigeon Pose

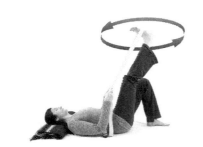

12. Hip Circles

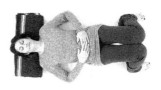

13. Reclined Leg Rest

SEQUENCE #11

Sequence for Core Strength

Gentle and Restorative Yoga (short sequence)

1. Practice **Reclined Leg Rest** for 5-10 minutes.
2. Grab your block and practice 10 rounds of **Bent Leg Abs With Block**. Repeat 2 more times. Pause between each round for slow belly breaths.
3. Place block between the thighs again and practice 10 rounds of **Bent Leg Twisting Abs with Block**. Repeat 2 more times. Pause between each round for slow belly breaths.
4. Remove the block and practice **Reclined Knee Hug (both knees)** for 10-20 slow cycles of breath.
5. Have your bolster ready and transition to **Supported Bridge With Bent Legs**. Slowly breathe for 3-5 minutes.
6. Release and practice **Pelvic Tilts** for 10-20 rounds.
7. Practice **Supported Final Relaxation** for 5-10 minutes.

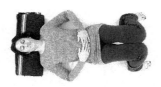
1. Reclined Leg Rest

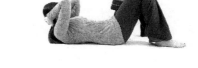
2. Bent Leg Abs with Block

SEQUENCE #11 (continued)

Sequence for Core Strength

Gentle and Restorative Yoga (short sequence)

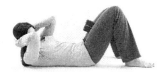

3. Bent Leg Twisting Abs with Block

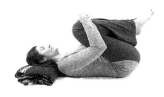

4. Reclined Knee Hug (both knees)

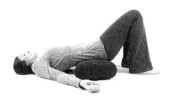

5. Supported Bridge with Bent Legs

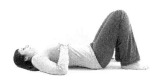

6. Pelvic Tilts

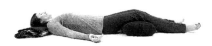

7. Supported Final Relaxation

SEQUENCE #12

Sequence for Core Strength

Gentle and Restorative Yoga (short sequence)

1. Practice **Reclined Knee Hug (both knees)** for 10-20 cycles of breath.
2. Keep the right knee hugged in and move into **Bicycle Abs** for 10 rounds. Release right knee and hug left in and practice 10 rounds.
3. Practice **Reclined Knee Hug (both knees)** for 10 slow breaths.
4. Practice **Bicycle Abs** for 10 more rounds each side.
5. Grab your block and practice 10 rounds of **Bent Leg Abs With Block**. Repeat 2 more times. Pause between each round for slow belly breaths.
6. Practice **Reclined Knee Hug (both knees)** for 5-10 cycles of breath.
7. Come onto one side, pause and then slowly transition into **Table Pose** and practice 5-10 rounds of **Cat/Cow Tilts**.
8. Move into **Plank Pose** and hold for 5-20 breaths.
9. Come into **Table Pose** and practice 5 more rounds of **Cat/Cow Tilts**.
10. Move into **Supported Belly Down Twist** and hold 6-8 minutes each side.
11. Practice **Supported Final Relaxation** for 5-10 minutes.

SEQUENCE #12 (continued)

Sequence for Core Strength
Gentle and Restorative Yoga (short sequence)

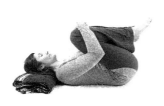

1. Reclined Knee Hug (both knees)

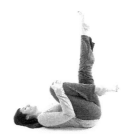

2. Bicycle Abs

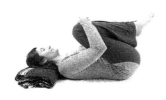

3. Reclined Knee Hug (both knees)

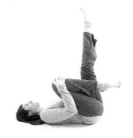

4. Bicycle Abs

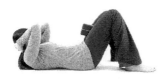

5. Bent Leg Abs with Block

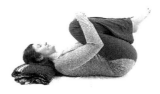

6. Reclined Knee Hug (both knees)

SEQUENCE #12 (continued)
Sequence for Core Strength
Gentle and Restorative Yoga (short sequence)

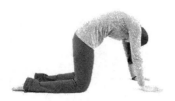

7. Cat/Cow Tilts

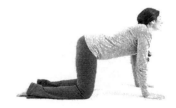

7. Cat/Cow Tilts

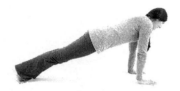

8. Plank Pose

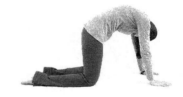

9. Cat/Cow Tilts

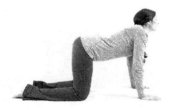

9. Cat/Cow Tilts

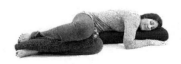

10. Supported Belly Down Twist

SEQUENCE #12 (continued)

Sequence for Core Strength

Gentle and Restorative Yoga (short sequence)

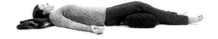

11. Supported Final Relaxation

SEQUENCE #13

Sequence for Core Strength

Gentle and Restorative Yoga (long sequence)

1. Come into **Table Pose** and practice 5-8 rounds of **Cat/Cow Tilts**.
2. From a neutral spine, move into **Table Extensions** for 10-20 breaths each side.
3. Pause and practice **Child's Pose** for 10-20 breaths.
4. Transition to **Plank Pose**. Hold for 5-20 breaths, lifting out of shoulders and engaging the core.
5. Come into **Table Pose** and practice 5-8 rounds of **Cat/Cow Tilts**.
6. From a neutral spine, move into **Supported Child's Pose**. Practice 3-4 minutes, turn the head, practice 3-4 more minutes.
7. Release **Supported Child's Pose** and practice **Modified Downward Facing Dog** or **Downward Facing Dog**, "walking the dog." Stretch until the back of the legs feel open.
8. Come onto the back and practice **Reclined Knee Hug (both knees)** for 10-20 cycles of breath.
9. Grab your block and practice 10 rounds of **Bent Leg Abs With Block**. Repeat 2 more times. Pause between each round for slow belly breaths.
10. Place block between the thighs again and practice 10 rounds of **Bent Leg Twisting Abs with Block**. Repeat 2 more times. Pause between each round for slow belly breaths.
11. Remove the block and practice **Reclined Knee Hug (both knees)** for 10-20 slow cycles of breath.
12. Move into **Supported Belly Down Twist** and hold 6-8 minutes each side.

SEQUENCE #13 (continued)

Sequence for Core Strength

Gentle and Restorative Yoga (long sequence)

13. Practice **Supported Final Relaxation** for 5-10 minutes.

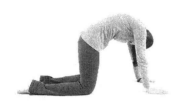

1. Cat/Cow Tilts

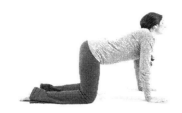

1. Cat/Cow Tilts

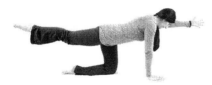

2. Table Extensions

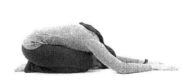

3. Child's Pose

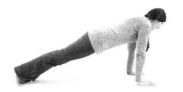

4. Plank Pose

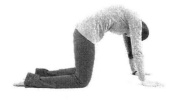

5. Cat/Cow Tilts

SEQUENCE #13 (continued)

Sequence for Core Strength
Gentle and Restorative Yoga (long sequence)

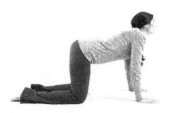

5. Cat/Cow Tilts

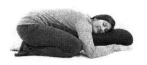

6. Supported Child's Pose

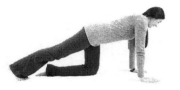

7. Modified Downward Facing Dog

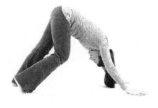

7. Downward Facing Dog (walking the dog)

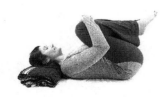

8. Reclined Knee Hug (both knees)

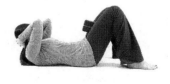

9. Bent Leg Abs with Block

SEQUENCE #13 (continued)

Sequence for Core Strength
Gentle and Restorative Yoga (long sequence)

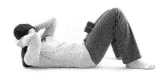
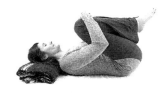

10. Bent Leg Twisting Abs with Block (right side)

11. Reclined Knee Hug (both knees)

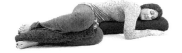
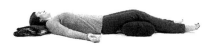

12. Supported Belly Down Twist

13. Supported Final Relaxation

SEQUENCE #14

Sequence for Core Strength

Gentle and Restorative Yoga (long sequence)

1. Grab your block and practice 10 rounds of **Bent Leg Abs With Block**. Repeat 2 more times. Pause between each round for slow belly breaths.
2. Practice **Reclined Leg Rest** for 5-10 minutes.
3. Release and practice **Reclined Knee Hug (both knees)** for 5-10 breaths.
4. Place block between the thighs again and practice 10 rounds of **Bent Leg Twisting Abs with Block**. Repeat 2 more times. Pause between each round for slow belly breaths.
5. Have your bolster ready and transition to **Supported Bridge With Bent Legs**. Slowly breathe for 3-5 minutes.
6. Release and practice **Pelvic Tilts** for 10-20 rounds.
7. Practice **Reclined Knee Hug (both knees)** for 10 slow breaths.
8. Hug right knee in and move into **Bicycle Abs** for 10 rounds. Release right knee and hug left in and practice 10 rounds.
9. Transition to **Reclined Knee Hug (both knees)** for 10 deep breaths.
10. Come into **Reclined Knee Down Twist** for 2-4 minutes each side.
11. Practice **Supported Final Relaxation** for 5-10 minutes.

SEQUENCE #14 (continued)

Sequence for Core Strength

Gentle and Restorative Yoga (long sequence)

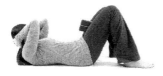

1. Bent Leg Abs with Block

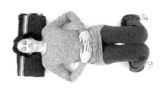

2. Reclined Leg Rest

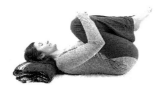

3. Reclined Knee Hug (both knees)

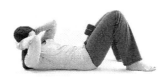

4. Bent Leg Twisting Abs with Block

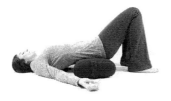

5. Supported Bridge with Bent Legs

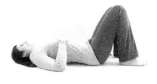

6. Pelvic Tilts

SEQUENCE #14 (continued)
Sequence for Core Strength
Gentle and Restorative Yoga (long sequence)

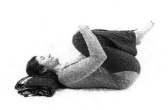

7. Reclined Knee Hug (both knees)

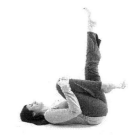

8. Bicycle Abs

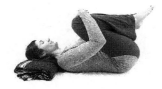

9. Reclined Knee Hug (both knees)

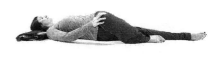

10. Reclined Knee Down Twist

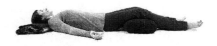

11. Supported Final Relaxation

SEQUENCE #15

Sequence for Core Strength

Gentle and Restorative Yoga (long sequence)

1. Come into **Table Pose** and practice 5-8 rounds of **Cat/Cow Tilts**.
2. From a neutral spine, move into **Supported Child's Pose**. Practice 3-4 minutes, turn the head, practice 3-4 more minutes.
3. Release **Supported Child's Pose** and practice **Modified Downward Facing Dog** or **Downward Facing Dog**, "walking the dog." Stretch until the back of the legs feel open.
4. From a neutral spine, move into **Table Extensions** for 10-20 breaths each side.
5. Come back to **Table Pose** and transition to **Child's Pose** for 10-20 cycles of breath.
6. Practice 5-8 rounds of **Cat/Cow Tilts**.
7. Transition into **Plank Pose** and breathe calmly for 5-20 cycles of breath while drawing the navel up to the spine.
8. Slowly come onto the belly for **Belly Down ½ Frog** and practice for 3-5 minutes each side.
9. Mindfully make your way onto the back for **Reclined Knee Hug (both knees)** for 10 cycles of breath.
10. Keep right knee hugged in and move into **Bicycle Abs** for 10 rounds. Release right knee and hug left in and practice 10 rounds.
11. Practice **Reclined Knee Hug (both knees)** for 5 slow breaths.
12. Move into **Reclined Knee Down Twist** for 3-5 minutes each side.
13. Practice **Supported Inversion** for 8-10 minutes.

SEQUENCE #15 (continued)
Sequence for Core Strength
Gentle and Restorative Yoga (long sequence)

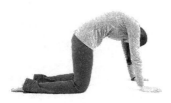

1. Cat/Cow Tilts

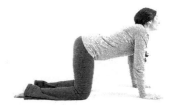

1. Cat/Cow Tilts

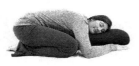

2. Supported Child's Pose

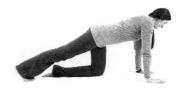

3. Modified Downward Facing Dog

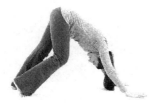

3. Downward Facing Dog (walking the dog)

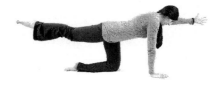

4. Table Extensions

SEQUENCE #15 (continued)

Sequence for Core Strength
Gentle and Restorative Yoga (long sequence)

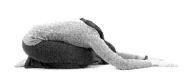

5. Child's Pose

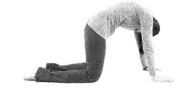

6. Cat/Cow Tilts

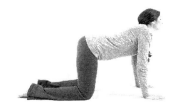

6. Cat/cow Tilts

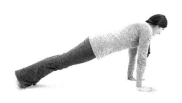

7. Plank Pose

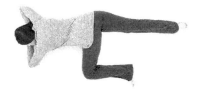

8. Belly Down ½ Frog

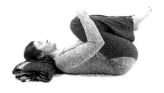

9. Reclined Knee Hug (both knees)

SEQUENCE #15 (continued)
Sequence for Core Strength
Gentle and Restorative Yoga (long sequence)

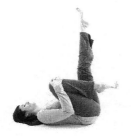

10. Bicycle Abs

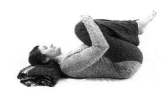

11. Reclined Knee Hug (both knees)

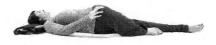

12. Reclined Knee Down Twist

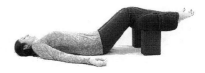

13. Supported Inversion

Inhale, peace and ease.
Exhale, tension and stress.
Thank you for allowing me to guide your practice.
May you walk with peace. Namaste.

Made in the USA
Columbia, SC
28 November 2018